Urban Health
In Developing Countries
Progress and Prospects

Edited by Trudy Harpham and Marcel Tanner

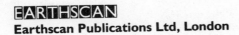
Earthscan Publications Ltd, London

First published in the UK in 1995 by
Earthscan Publications Limited

A catalogue record for this book is available from the British Library

ISBN: 1 85383 285 5 (HB)
ISBN: 1 85383 281 2 (PB)

Typesetting and figures by PCS Mapping & DTP, Newcastle upon Tyne

Printed and bound by Biddles Ltd, Guildford and Kings Lynn

Cover design by Dominic Banner

Cover photo courtesy of

For a full list of publications please contact:
Earthscan Publications Limited
120 Pentonville Road
London N1 9JN
Tel. (0171) 278 0433
Fax: (0171) 278 1142

Earthscan is an editorially independent subsidiary of Kogan Page Limited and
publishes in association with WWF-UK and the International Institute for
Environment and Development.

Contents

List of Illustrations

List of Contributors

SARAH ATKINSON Lecturer, Geography Department, Mansfield Cooper Building, University of Manchester, Oxford Road, Manchester M13 9PL, UK

CHRISTIAN AUER Epidemiologist c/o Servants, PO Box AC569, 1109 Quezon City, Cubao, Philippines

ANTOINE DEGRÉMONT Professor and Director, Swiss Tropical Institute, Socinstrasse 57, PO Box 4002, Basel, Switzerland

MARIA ELENA DUCCI Instituto de Estudios Urbanos, Universidad Católica de Chile, El Comendador 1916, Casilla 16002, Santiago 9, Chile

MICHAEL DUNCAN Programme Coordinator c/o Servants, PO Box AC569, 1109 Quezon City, Cubao, Philippines

QUAZI GHIASUDDIN Deputy Director, Save the Children Fund (UK), Bangladesh

DOREEN GIHANGA Coordinator, Kampala MCH Project, Save the Children Fund (UK), Uganda

LILIA DURAN GONZALEZ Director, Nuredess - Xalapa, National Institute of Public Health, Tuxpan 18, Fraccionamiento Veracruz, CP 91020, Xalapa, VER. Mexico

HOLLY FLUTY Office of Health, US Agency for International Development, SA18 Room 1266, Department of State, Washington DC 20523-1817, USA

PAUL GARNER Senior Lecturer, International Health Division, Liverpool School of Tropical Medicine, Pembroke Place, Liverpool L3 5QA, UK

GREG GOLDSTEIN Responsible Officer, Environmental Health, World Health Organization, Avenue Appia, 1211 Geneva 27, Switzerland

TRUDY HARPHAM Professor, School of Urban Policy, South Bank University, Wandsworth Road, London SW8 2JZ, UK

ROBERT HECHT Senior Principal, The World Bank, Room T-7107, 1818H Street NW, Washington DC 20433, USA

EMILE JEANNÉE Programme Director in Chad, Department of Public Health and Epidemiology, Swiss Tropical Institute, Socinstrasse 57, PO Box 4002, Basel, Switzerland

KATHERINE KAYE Epidemiologist, Health Unit, Save the Children USA, 54 Wilton Road, Westport, Connecticut 06880, USA

MATTHIAS KERKER Scientific Advisor, Human Resources/Health, Swiss Development Cooperation, Eigerstrasse 73, 3003 Bern Switzerland

PETER KILIMA Deputy City Medical Officer of Health and Co-Project Manager, Dar-es-Salaam Urban Health Project, PO Box 63320, Dar es Salaam, Tanzania

ULI KNOBLOCH Consultant, Proyecto APS/NORSSALUD-GTZ, AP 2365, Cúcuta, Colombia

JENNIFER LISSFELT Senior Research Associate, The Futures Group International, 1050th Street NW, Washington DC 20036, USA

NICK LORENZ Programme Director, Dar es Salaam Urban Health Project, Department of Public Health and Epidemiology, Swiss Tropical Institute, Socinstrasse 57, PO Box 4002, Basel, Switzerland

BARBARA MCPAKE Lecturer, Health Economics and Financing Programme, Department of Public Health and Policy, London School of Hygiene and Tropical Medicine, Keppel Street, London WC1E 7HT, UK

FRED MERKLE Senior Planning Specialist, Health, Population, Nutrition, GTZ, PO Box 5180, 65726 Eschborn, Germany

MIKE O'DWYER Regional Health Adviser, Save the Children Fund, (UK), East Africa Regional Office, Kenya

R PADMINI Senior Urban Adviser, UNICEF, DH-40E, 3 UN Plaza, New York, NY 10017, USA

NGUDUP PALJOR Project Director, Urban Health Extension Project, International Centre for Diarrhoeal Disease Research, Bangladesh (ICDDR,B) GPO Box 128, Dhaka 1000, Bangladesh

VOAHANGY N RAMAHATAFANDRY Technical Advisor, Medical Component of the PADS Project, Swiss Tropical Institute, BP 972, N'Djamena, Chad

ALESSANDRO ROSSI-ESPAGNET Consultant, World Health Organization, Avenue Appia, 1211 Geneva 27, Switzerland

JOHN SEAGER Head, National Urbanization and Health Research Programme, Medical Research Council, PO Box 19070, Tygerberg 7505, South Africa

DIANA SILIMPERI Senior Program Associate, Strengthening Health Services Program, Management Sciences for Health, 165 Allandale Road, Boston MA 12130, USA

IRAJ TABIBZADEH Responsible Officer, District Health Systems, Division of Strengthening Health Services, World Health Organization, Avenue Appia, 1211 Geneva 27, Switzerland

MARCEL TANNER Professor and Head, Department of Public Health and Epidemiology, Swiss Tropical Institute, Socinstrasse 57, PO Box 4002, Basel, Switzerland

MARGARET THOMAS Consultant Health Economist for Developing Countries, 108A Settrington Road, London SW6 3BA, UK

GUSTAVO TORRES Urban Planner, Consultant Urban Development, Virgen del Puerto 9, Madrid 28005, Spain

C ASHOK KUMAR YESUDIAN Professor and Head, Dept of Health Services Studies, Tata Institute of Social Sciences, Sion-Trombay Road, Deonar, Bombay 400088, India

Preface

The idea of this book originated at the 'Urban Health Consultation' which was held in Eggiwil, Switzerland in late 1992 as part of the preparations for the World Bank's *World Development Report 1993 – Investing in Health*. The Consultation was organized by the Swiss Tropical Institute and the London School of Hygiene and Tropical Medicine and was funded by the Swiss Development Corporation and the Swiss Tropical Institute.

The participants of the Consultation felt that the wealth of important and interesting information presented and discussed merited the publication of a book to disseminate the material more widely. Specially commissioned chapters complement this material and are presented here in order to highlight initiatives in urban health development since the late 1980s when the last comprehensive review on this subject was published. The views and case studies are necessarily selective and particular emphasis has been given to the role of multilateral and bilateral agencies as well as nongovernmental organizations in supporting urban health in developing countries. The editors are aware that numerous initiatives at city level in particular countries could not be given a platform here although several of them are referred to in the introductory and concluding chapters.

In addition to acknowledging all the efforts of the contributors, editors and authors who have made this book possible, we would like to thank Vanessa Lavender and Jane Pelerin for their skilful editorial assistance and Jennifer Jenkins for critically reviewing a number of manuscripts. Christine Walliser provided valuable secretarial support during the whole preparation of the book. We are in debt to our publishers, Earthscan, for the patience they have demonstrated during the realization of the project. Professor Harpham's participation was made possible by the UK Overseas Development Administration's funding of the Urban Health Programme at the London School of Hygiene and Tropical Medicine.

We hope and expect that urban health issues will be on more agendas in the future and that this book will contribute to people's understanding of the current trends, may stimulate the implementation of urban health programmes and generate relevant research projects.

Trudy Harpham and Marcel Tanner, London 1995

Glossary

ARI	Acute Respiratory Infections
CDR	Control of Diarrhoeal and Respiratory Diseases (Programme)
DALY	Disability Adjusted Life Year
ENHR	Essential National Health Research
EPI	Expanded Programme on Immunization
FAO	Food and Agricultural Organization
FP	Family Planning
HABITAT	United Nations Centre for Human Settlements
IEC	Information, Education and Communication
MCH	Mother and Child Health/Maternal and Child Health
MOH	Ministry of Health
NGO	Nongovernmental Organization
ODA	Overseas Development Administration (UK)
PHC	Primary Health Care
PVO	Private Voluntary Organization
SAP	Structural Adjustment Programme
SDC	Swiss Development Corporation
SHS	Strengthening Health Services
STI	Swiss Tropical Institute
UBS	Urban Basic Services
UCI	Universal Childhood Immunization
UNICEF	United Nations Children's Fund
USAID	United States Agency for International Development
WHO	World Health Organization

1

Urbanization and Health in Developing Countries – a Review of Some Trends

Trudy Harpham and Marcel Tanner

Cities are the locus of productive economic activities and hope for the future, yet they face growing environmental problems and increasing poverty'... 'It is clear that, in the short term, the bright lights of the city have dimmed and are, for many urban households, extinguished.

(World Bank 1991)

Urbanization... will become one of the most critical development issues in the years ahead. Lynda Chalker, Minister of Overseas Development, UK

(Harris 1992)

INTRODUCTION

Since the publication of the first two books on urban health in developing countries (*In the shadow of the city: community health in the urban poor* by Harpham (ed) et al 1988 and *Spotlight on the cities* by Tabibzadeh et al 1989) there have been a number of shifts on the part of international agencies with regard to their policy towards urban health development. There have also been a number of interesting programme development activities within countries and the production of additional information on health status among low income urban populations. This chapter highlights a selection of trends which both point to the direction of future developments and link to chapters in this book.

The chapter is divided into two sections: initiatives arising in the health sector and initiatives arising in the urban sector. While this division is somewhat artificially contrived it nonetheless reflects the reality that individuals working on health projects and programmes attempting to address urban specific issues often know little about what their colleagues in the urban sector are doing and *vice versa*. Indeed, one of the issues for the late 1990s and the 21st century is to enable these two sectors to interact more closely and to draw lessons from each other. The very definition of the 'urban sector' itself causes problems which are addressed below. The demographics of urbanization in developing countries are not rehearsed here as there is now an abundance of texts and articles on the phenomenon (for example, see Drakakis-Smith 1987 and Palen 1992). Similarly, it is not the intention of this book to repeat descriptions of urban health problems which can be found in other, recent texts, although highlights of selected studies are briefly discussed.

URBAN ISSUES IN THE HEALTH SECTOR

Multilateral organizations

The two multilateral organizations which have explicit objectives to improve health are the World Health Organization (WHO) and UNICEF. The chapters by Goldstein et al and Padmini document the support that these two organizations have provided to urban health initiatives. Taking a wider look at the activities of the two organizations one can discern in both of them a struggle to deal with the need to consider broader issues when dealing with urban health. In WHO the Healthy Cities Project is unique because of its inter-programmatic function. However, this attribute might also explain the fact that the project has been criticized for 'its lack of overt progress and measurable impact' (Silimperi 1994, p 13). Although an urban health committee was established with members from the Control of Diarrhoeal and Respiratory Diseases Programme (CDR), the Expanded Programme on Immunization (now the Global Vaccination Programme), Strengthening Health Services (SHS), and Environmental Health Division, most initiatives remain specific to the separate divisions (at the time of writing, the Healthy Cities Project initiative is still firmly within the Environmental Health Division). However, the Healthy Cities Project is now receiving an increasing amount of attention from bilateral funders and is likely to take off in the next few years (with, for example, the possibility of the Dutch government funding the project in numerous cities).

Turning to UNICEF, the Urban Basic Services (UBS) Programme (see the chapter by Padmini) finds itself at a crisis point and has recently undergone institutional scrutiny. A meeting of 'urban experts' was called in late 1993 to examine UNICEF's new urban policy and to assess the future direction of UBS. During the meeting the issue of evaluation of UBS was often raised. While UBS has a fine tradition of community development work it has not always been able to demonstrate achievement in terms of UNICEF's mid-decade and summit goals. In other words, it is rare to find impact measures of success for UBS in documents. It is ironic that the Urban Basic Services Programme appears to be under threat from the headquarters of UNICEF while at the national level it is being adopted by national governments as a way forward for urban development in general. In India for example, UBS is pivotal in the future national urban development programme which is attempting to replicate the UBS approach across whole states such as Andhra Pradesh. Indeed, arguments are being presented to bilateral funders, like the UK Overseas Development Administration (ODA), that they should move away from their support for Slum Improvement Projects in India to supporting Urban Basic Services nationally, which might lead their aid to be more sustainable and replicable (see Harpham and Stephens 1992 for a discussion of the strengths and weaknesses of the slum improvement approach).

Bilateral and Non-governmental organizations

The early 1990s witnessed a growing number of urban health initiatives as integral parts of national health sector reform efforts. For example, the UK ODA support of health sector reform in Zambia includes an urban health project in Lusaka which will strengthen the role of urban health centres *vis à vis* the hospital, facilitate community involvement in health councils, improve the management capacity of the city health department etc. ODA supports a similar project in Lahore within the 'Second Pakistan Family Health Project'. Other European bilaterals are convinced of the importance of supporting urban health development, for example the German technical agency GTZ (see the chapter by Merkle and Knobloch) and the Swiss Development Corporation (SDC). SDC started its interest in urban health on the basis of its health sector policy. Least developed countries, high risk groups of the population and the implementation of primary health care are basic guiding principles of the policy. With regard to implementation strategies, SDC emphasizes the health district management approach (reviewed in Lorenz et al 1994). It is in this context that SDC also paid attention to the development of cities in selected countries, namely the Republic of Chad and Tanzania. The urban health components for the cities of Dar es Salaam, Tanzania, and N'Djamena, Republic of Chad, were initiated in 1989 when the World Bank designed the structural adjustment programmes (SAP) for these countries. In the Republic of Chad, SDC co-financed the SAP and targeted its funds to the urban health component for N'Djamena. The Swiss Tropical Institute (STI), on behalf of the Chadian and Swiss governments, became responsible for the technical assistance of the urban health component. Consequently the urban health component became well integrated into the overall health development approach of the Préfecture of Chari Baguirmi (of which the city of N'Djamena is part) for which STI was already responsible as part of a bilateral agreement between Switzerland and the Republic of Chad.

In Tanzania, the urban health project is implemented under a bilateral agreement between Switzerland and Tanzania. The project is funded by SDC, and STI acts as the executing agency on behalf of both governments. The project aims at the structural and functional rehabilitation of the governmental health care delivery and health promotion services. After a preparation phase of nearly two years, it started in late 1990 and initially emphasized structural rehabilitation. This phase was soon followed by a strong emphasis on community involvement, assisting local initiatives and health promotion activities.

SDC pursues in both urban health 'projects' a programme-based approach that consists of assisting the regional health authorities to plan and implement health development activities within the concept of health district management. Strong emphasis is placed on implementing primary health care principles and comprehensive district health plans. Given the nature and concept of SDC's support for urban health, it is evident that SDC has a long-term commitment, up to ten years, to supporting health development in the metropolitan areas of these countries.

Turning to another bilateral, Fluty and Lissfelt's chapter provides an account of the rising interest in urban health within the United States Agency for International Development (USAID) and emphasizes that a particular strategy is needed because most of the problems and opportunities arising from urbanization cross USAID's sectoral and programme boundaries. This is a problem which an increasing number of agencies are facing and it will be interesting to observe which agencies tackle the challenge with imagination and which retreat into the secure, traditional sectoral divisions.

International Non-governmental organizations (NGOs) have an increasingly important role in urban health development as reflected in the chapter by Atkinson (ed) and as evidenced by the pioneering efforts in this field by groups such as Oxfam (UK) which supported the first international meeting on urban health back in 1984. New actors on the scene include the Rockefeller Foundation which is identifying challenges for urban health in the 21st century. No case studies of Third World NGOs are given here but an excellent, recent publication (Arrossi et al 1994) presents 18 case studies of intermediary institutions (most of them Third World NGOs) who provide technical, legal and financial services to low-income urban households for improving housing, sanitation, drainage, health care and other community services (see also Hardoy et al 1990). The case studies demonstrated

> that there are ways to address poverty successfully, without large subsidies. The methods used in the case studies are generally far more cost-effective than those of traditional development projects which tend to have a relatively small impact in relation to the scale of investment... [and]... demonstrate that intermediary institutions can provide support for individual and community initiatives in which poorer groups and their community organizations retain control of what is done and how it is done.

(Arrossi et al 1994 p70)

A changing urban health profile

In addition to changes in the level of interest in supporting urban health initiatives in the last decade there has also been more information made available about the extent and types of urban health problems. A sufficient number of descriptive studies have documented that the urban poor suffer the worst of both worlds – infectious disease and malnutrition from underdevelopment and chronic diseases from modernization (Harpham et al 1988, Songsore and McGranahan 1993, Pryer 1993, Surjadi 1993 and Satterthwaite 1993). Just as in the North where the epidemiological transition saw the so-called 'diseases of affluence' transformed into the diseases of the poor, in the South we also begin to see coronary heart disease, stroke and obesity becoming more common among the least well off (Wilkinson 1994). This pattern is most evident in urban areas (Stephens et al 1994). The increasing importance of psychosocial health problems in low-income urban areas of the South has also been recently documented (Harpham 1994). It is now time to turn to studies which assess the cost-effectiveness of interventions against 'the new urban killers' (see below and the chapter by Seager).

HEALTH ISSUES IN THE URBAN SECTOR

Until recently few aid agencies gave much support to city or municipal governments to improve urban health. Many of the recent initiatives in urban health are strongly project based, as reflected in the descriptions of the activities of bilateral and multilateral donors in many countries of the developing world (see the chapters by Goldstein et al, Padmini, Hecht, Fluty and Lissfelt, and Merkle and Knobloch). These projects are often not very well integrated into the existing health care delivery and health promotion system of the countries concerned and/or do not pursue the health district management approach. Reviewing the chapters that describe the various initiatives of these donors as well as NGOs reveals the strong relationship of the projects and programmes with the respective Ministries of Health. However, any Ministry of Health is mainly a technical ministry that has little control of overall planning activities at central and local government levels. One might therefore argue, and this is reflected in the conclusions of the chapter on determinants (Tanner and Harpham), that future approaches should reduce the degree of medicalization of urban health projects and no longer rely to such a large extent on Ministries of Health, but finalize the implementation arrangements with Ministries of Local Government and municipalities.

Hardoy and Satterthwaite (1992) have analyzed multilateral agencies' (mainly the development associations and banks) expenditure on water supply and sanitation, the improvement of shelter, primary health care and primary education and literacy programmes. Most agencies dedicated less than 10 per cent of their total commitments to these inputs. UNICEF, with its emphasis on Urban Basic Services was a notable exception. Most expenditure in the urban sector was on large infrastructure projects such as ports, power stations and public transport. For bilaterals, these investments promote their exports and contracts for their own companies.

The World Bank began a programme of support to urban projects in 1972 and is now the largest single donor for urban projects (Hardoy and Satterthwaite 1992). Funds are still small in relation to needs and there is now a trend to move away from support for projects such as sites and services, slum upgrading, towards strengthening city and municipal governments to manage urban development. Stren (1989) has termed this the 'management' approach to urban reform. The Urban Management Programme, a joint initiative of UNDP, the World Bank and the United

Nations Centre for Human Settlements (HABITAT) provides technical assistance for building institutional capacity. This move from projectized support to policy analysis and institutional development is reflected in the Bank's urban agenda for the 1990s (World Bank 1991) and resulted from the failure to achieve citywide impacts from neighbourhood-based projects. The policy framework which is suggested for the 1990s includes moving towards a broader view of urban issues (ie wider than the housing sector) and enhancing the productivity of the urban poor by improving access to social services. Both of these changes suggest that urban health will become a central issue. The Bank's support of urban health development is further analyzed in the chapter by Hecht.

The new urban policy of the Bank focuses on increasing the productivity of the urban economy in order to strengthen the national macro-economic position. Ironically, it is noted that urban poverty is a particular problem in countries which have agreed to structural adjustment as advocated by the World Bank. This is because: the urban poor are dependent upon their labour, rather than asset ownership, so are particularly affected by rising unemployment; the cuts in public expenditure (for example on health), which are part of structural adjustment, tend to have a disproportionate impact on the poor; and changes in tariffs and subsidies with resulting rising prices affect the urban poor, who are dependent upon a cash economy, more than their rural counterparts (World Bank 1991). The new policy advocates increasing social sector expenditure on basic services but does not reconcile this with the cuts in social sector expenditure required in structural adjustment. There is increasing evidence that, contrary to the World Bank predictions that the urban informal sector will thrive under free market conditions, the informal sector has in fact been squeezed from both the supply and the demand side. On the supply side, raw materials are scarce due to formal industrial producers now recycling waste products which were previously inputs of informal producers. On the demand side, the substantial contraction in demand among low income wage earners who normally purchase goods and services from informal producers has had a particularly strong negative effect.*

The new World Bank (1991) policy also gives research a prominent role. It is argued that there has been a decline in urban research capacity just when many urban policy questions are becoming increasingly important. 'The need is thus great for increasing research on urban issues' (p12). Interestingly the decline in urban development research has been in parallel with a growth in urban health research (see Seager's chapter). One suggested priority area for research is the role of government in the urban development process. This is particularly welcome as, from the health perspective, it is now crucial to examine the role of municipalities in the development of urban health. In particular, the division of resources and responsibilities between central and local governments needs comparative analysis to identify the most successful approaches for particular contexts.

The agenda for priority research is still very large. There is definitely

---

* Based on a study in Zaria, Nigeria by Meagher and Yunusa 1991

a need to design more analytical studies, as the first decades of urban health research have provided the crucial descriptive elements, pointed out the high risk areas and groups and have generated a substantial number of hypotheses. Analytical approaches require a different type of research design. Besides intervention studies, community based action research will be required to monitor social development in urban areas and to elucidate its determinants. This is also indicated in the Seager chapter which summarizes the evolution and current issues for urban health research. One recent development which is bound to affect the future direction of urban health research is the development of particular methods used in the first *World Development Report* to focus on health. Murray et al (1994) propose disability adjusted life years (DALYs) as a comparable measure of disease burden. DALYs were used as one important basis of the *World Development Report 1993* (World Bank 1993) which revealed that urban areas carry about one quarter of the global burden of disease. This not only points to the need to focus on health development in urban areas, but also raises demand for a non-disease DALY concept. Given the substantial interdependencies of diseases with sociocultural and socioeconomic factors, risk based DALYs would help to establish more appropriately the burden of ill-health in urban areas as well as priority areas of intervention.

MULTISECTOR BOOK

In true reflection of the multisector nature of urban health development the following chapters are contributed by both health and urban development specialists who are trying to work together to share their respective lessons and knowledge. This is even evident in the editorship which has been performed by a Professor of Public Health and a Professor of Urban Development. The contributions also represent a balance between implementers and researchers and between writers from the South and the North (although most of the editing has been done by academics from the North). This mixture is important, as Donabedian (1986) states: '...The world of ideas and the world of action are not separate... but inseparable parts of each other. Ideas in particular, are truly pointed forces that shape the tangible world. The man and woman of action have no less responsibility to know and understand than does the scholar...'

REFERENCES

Arrossi, S Bombarolo, F Hardoy, J Mitlin, D Coscio, L and Satterthwaite, D (1994) *Funding Community Initiatives: the Role of NGOs and Other Intermediary Institutions in Supporting Low Income Groups and Their Community Organizations in Improving Housing and Living Conditions in the Third World* Earthscan, London

Donabedian, (1986) The Baxter American Foundation Prize Address *Journal of Health Administration*, 4, pp611–614

Drakakis-Smith, D (1987) *The Third World City* Methuen, London

Hardoy, J and Satterthwaite, D (1992) *Environmental Problems in Third World Cities: an Agenda for the Poor and the Planet* International Institute for Environment and

Development, London

Hardoy, J, Cairncross, S, and Satterthwaite, D (eds) (1990) *The Poor Die Young: Housing and Health in Third World Cities* Earthscan, London

Harpham, T and Pepperall, J (1994) 'Planning Decentralization of Urban Health Activities in Developing Countries' *Development in Practice*, 4 (2), pp92–99

Harpham, T (1994) 'Urbanization and Mental Health in Developing Countries: Research Role for Social Scientists, Public Health Professionals and Social Psychiatrists' *Social Science and Medicine*, 39 (2), pp233–245

Harpham, T and Stephens, C (1992) 'Policy Directions in Urban Health in Developing Countries – the Slum Improvement Approach' *Social Science and Medicine*, 35 (2), pp111–120

Harpham, T Lusty, T and Vaughan, P (1988) *In the Shadow of the City: Community Health and the Urban Poor* Oxford University Press, Oxford

Harris, N (1992) *Cities in the 1990s: the Challenge for Developing Countries* UCL Press, London

Lorenz, N, Burnier, E and Tanner, M (1994) 'Schweizerische Unterstützung von Distriktsgesundheitssystemen in Entwicklungsländern' *Jahrbuch Schweiz – Dritte Welt*, 13, pp185–205

Meagher, K and Yunusa, M (1991) *Limits to Labour Absorption: Conceptual and Historical Background to Adjustment in Nigeria's Urban Informal Economy*. Discussion paper no 28. United Nations Research Institution for Social Development, Geneva

Murray, C and Lopez, A (1994) 'The Global Burden of Disease in 1990: Summary Results, Sensitivity Analysis and Future Directions' *Bulletin of the World Health Organization'* 72 (3), pp495–509

Palen, J (1992) *The Urban World* McGraw-Hill, New York

Pryer, J (1993) 'The Impact of Adult Ill Health on Household Income and Nutrition in Khula, Bangladesh' *Environment and Urbanization*, 5 (2), pp35–49

Satterthwaite, D (1993) 'The Impact on Health of Urban Environment' *Environment and Urbanization*, 5(2), pp87–111

Silimperi (1994) 'Delivering Child Survival Services to High Risk Populations' Unpublished paper for USAID's 'BASICS' project

Songsore, J and McGranahan, G (1993) 'Environment, Wealth and Health: Towards an Analysis of Intra-urban Differentials within Greater Accra Metropolitan Area, Ghana' *Environment and Urbanization*, 5, (2) pp10–34

Stephens, C Timaeus, I Akerman, M Ayle, S Maia, P Campanario, P Doe, B Lush, L Tettch, D Harpham, T (1994) *Environment and Health in Developing Countries: an Analysis of Intra-Urban Differentials Using Existing Data* Unpublished monograph. London School of Hygiene and Tropical Medicine.

Stren, R (1989) 'Urban Local Government in Africa' in Stren, R and White, R (eds) *African Cities in Crisis* Westview Press, London

Surjadi, C (1993) 'Respiratory Diseases of Mothers and Children and Environmental Factors among Households in Jakarta' *Environment and Urbanization*, 5 (2) pp78–86

Tabibzadeh, I, A Rossi-Espagnet (1989) *Spotlight on the cities: Improving urban health in developing countries* World Health Organisation, Geneva

Wilkinson, R (1994) 'The Epidemiological Transition: from Material Scarcity to Social Disadvantage?' Daedalus (*Journal of the American Academy of Arts and Sciences*) 123, pp61–78

World Bank (1991) *Urban Policy and Economic Development: an Agenda for the 1990s* World Bank, Washington DC

World Bank (1993) *World Development Report 1993 – Investing in Health* Oxford University Press, Oxford

2

Linkages for Urban Health – the Community and Agencies

Diana R Silimperi

INTRODUCTION

T he focus of this chapter is urban community participation in the delivery of community based primary health and family planning services (including preventive, public health and/or curative services). A framework for mobilizing urban communities will be presented as well as several essential principles and tools for strengthening community capacity to facilitate linkages between community members, health providers and agencies that provide services which normally lie outside the traditional health sector, but which significantly influence the health status of a community ('healthy connections').* Finally, selected examples of 'vehicles' for mobilizing and improving urban community-based health services are discussed.

Defining the urban community

A first critical step in mobilizing community participation is determining the definition and identity of the urban community; practically speaking, what is an urban 'community'? Is the community defined by administrative or jurisdictional borders, by demarcations for the provision of public services or geographic boundaries? How do legal, political or administrative delineations of community compare with the members' own sense of identity and placement of its communal borders? Given the heterogeneity and mobility of urban dwellers, it is not surprising that individuals living in urban settlements have been reported to have a diminished sense of community (Rifkin 1987); however, it may also be that multiple, often conflicting, delineations by political and administrative systems make it more difficult for an

---

* The term 'healthy connections' is used with permission from The Healthy Connections Programme at Children's Hospital in Boston

individual to identify or describe a community. In addition, it is possible that new and diverse definitions of community (and concomitant borders) have developed in urban settings, which are not so easily discerned by the non-community member (in contrast to rural areas where geographic or physical limits more clearly define the borders of most communities).

The word 'community' has several usages. In urban settings, more than in rural ones, there may be several concurrent 'functional' definitions of community: community may be defined according to geographic limits associated with administrative responsibilities for public services or governance; by physical borders which clearly divide areas (rivers or bodies of water, major highways, etc), or by a likeness of physical structures such as similar or connected housing. But, it may also be defined by shared characteristics, cultural traditions or functions of individual members, who may not be living in geographic proximity to each other (Loewy 1987 and Rifkin et al 1988). In general, urban planners and health agencies have utilized public service or governance delineations to distinguish community borders. However, if these borders do not coincide with the community's own functional identity based on shared characteristics or vision, attempts to promote community participation in health services cannot succeed. Such diversity in community definition and associated identity must be understood in the context of an urban setting before one can begin to address the roles a community plays or its participation in health promotion and services.

Let us first examine the former definition: the formal delineations of community as designated by or for governance (political) or the administration of public services. In most cities (and for the purposes of this chapter, we will use the word 'cities' to mean settlements over approximately 100,000 inhabitants), one finds that the public service or administrative designations are subject to frequent change according to political decisions or alterations in political power at the municipal, state or provincial level. Furthermore, over the last decade, as many governments pursued policies of decentralization, the power of urban authorities and their borders of jurisdictions – in terms of human and capital resource allocation, decision making authority and the literal provision of social/health services – has been in continuous flux (Rakowski and Kastner 1985 and Rossi-Espagnet 1983).

In addition, the changing physical configuration of a city due to, for example, population shifts, natural disasters or industrialization also results in the formation of new geographic community borders. Cities are dynamic structures; not only do they change in terms of the number of inhabitants, but also in terms of their shape as they 'consume' surrounding territories, reclaim or destroy internal sections for industrial development. These significant shifts in subpopulations affect intra-urban, residential population densities and consequently may alter the delineations of community borders for public services and governance.

Furthermore, even within one geographic urban community there may be varying boundaries for different types of public services, and the service borders may not coincide with the political or administrative units created for the purpose of governance. For example, a community's borders for the delivery of municipal health services are seldom the same as those determining its limits for schools, police services, water supply or garbage collection. This multiplicity of designated community service borders makes it difficult for urban citizens, especially new immigrants, to effectively mobilize needed services, or to obtain maximal assistance at the local level. Hence, the reported lack of urban community identity or participation may be related to a complicated environment which necessitates sophisticated knowledge regarding administrative boundaries and jurisdictions. Many urban dwellers need assistance to better understand overall municipal boundaries, as well as intra-urban borders which create geographic communities for the purpose of delivering public services (and associated resource allocation). They must also learn the titles and names of the specific individuals with designated responsibility for various services in their community (however it is defined).

The enlightened urban community member must also have a clear understanding of municipal versus provincial or state responsibilities for urban services, and be able to define these responsibilities in terms of decision making power and authority over resources in contrast to responsibility for supervision and implementation of the services. Mapping the borders of authority and power versus service implementation responsibility is an extremely useful activity, which can help one understand the relationship of power, governance and service. Mapping also graphically depicts overlapping jurisdictions and/or gaps in jurisdiction that may arise between departments or between municipal and state agencies in a rapidly changing urban environment. Such an exercise is useful not only for the community, but also for those responsible for delivering the services! One problem which such mapping powerfully illustrates is the lack of responsibility to provide health and related services in the so-called informal or peri-urban settlements, noted by different terms in various cultures, but all referring to those settlements of a city that are not formally recognized by the legal or governing authorities to be 'legitimate' urban communities, deserving of services and resources (Management Sciences for Health, FPMD 1992).

Although it is important for urban dwellers to have a clear understanding of the political and service borders of their community in order to more effectively mobilize or coordinate services, nonetheless many urban inhabitants may not define their community according to either geographic or administrative borders. Over the last decade, community development and health workers have frequently decried the weakened or splintered sense of community among urban dwellers, and the resultant increase in time and energy required to initiate community development or participatory health projects (Rifkin 1987). Certainly a weakened community identity is not surprising if one considers the mobility (intra-urban and rural to urban) of many urban families, the breakdown of traditional family structures and changing gender roles, and the ethnic and sociocultural diversity prevalent in most cities (Silimperi 1994).

However, more recently, there appears to be an emerging awareness among those working in cities that an urban 'community' identity does exist, although variations in this phenomenon may occur between cities. Nonetheless, recognition of this community identity by outsiders may be more difficult, since the foundation of such an urban community identity may not conform to geographic proximity or easily discerned political and administrative boundaries. One urban community may define itself along ethnic, cultural or linguistic similarities (for example new urban immigrants from the same village, tribe or country commonly seen in Asian and African cities such as Karachi or Nairobi); another may forge a new identity based on common environmental problems which threaten all members such as violence, pollution or the lack of solid waste disposal; and yet a third identity may be dependent upon common function or workplace (garment or factory workers in Dhaka or daily labourers in urban India). In cities more than in rural areas, community identity may also be defined in terms of employment function or location since so many hours are spent away from one's residence. Adults with children will often identify their community in terms of school or related recreational and social networks.

None of these examples negate the fact that some urban communities may still use geographic proximity as a source of community identification, but only serve to emphasize the fact that diverse definitions exist for urban communities, including new meanings based on common function or characteristics, in addition to geography and physical borders. (In rural areas, the lack of diversity within most communities results in a less dominant role of shared characteristics in the formation of community identity; or when differences in such characteristics exist, they often coincide with differences in geography.)

One particular characteristic which deserves special mention is duration of urban residence. New migrants to the cities may continue to identify with their community of origin and its habits, but within one or two generations the identity of the new urban community has been adopted.

Because the borders of urban communities are both fluid and diverse, and may not conform simply to geographic proximity or governing boundaries, as well as the fact that many urban communities have sociocultural norms or languages which vary from those of the health service provider or community development organizer, a range of misperceptions about the strength of urban communities may have been perpetuated without intent. On the other hand, it is also clear that urban populations are dynamic, and that the very definition of community has and is changing in many cities. More study is necessary to better understand these emerging configurations and definitions of community in urban settings, and the changes that take place as a city matures in size and space, and as its residents become long term urban dwellers. Such study will illuminate new ways to reach, mobilize and serve urban communities. In the meantime, understanding the identity and definition of an urban community is the first prerequisite to mobilization.

Selecting the type of community participation: matching community characteristics and participation type

The second step in mobilization is to analyze the type of participation most appropriate and suited to the characteristics of the community. Too often the term 'community participation' has been used in a constricting fashion, referring merely to financial or in-kind resource contribution for a health service or facility, or to literal participation in the delivery of services through community members who function as providers. Particularly in cities, diverse types of participation are possible. Box 2.1 describes several possible types of community participation. For example, one type may be financial support; individual members of the community or a community organization provide direct monetary or in-kind compensation for the provision of health services, thereby subsidizing the salaries of the providers and other operational costs of the facility. Another type of participation may be community management or administrative responsibility for the implementation of health services, which could but doesn't necessarily include overall decision making authority regarding the health services or providers. Because many urban, community based health services are dependent upon external donors for financial, technical and administrative support, it is rare that full decision making authority is based in the community.

Individual or organized group advocacy for the community's perceived needs, especially with external authorities or agencies responsible for the provision of services, is yet another critical type of community participation. Finally, the direct contribution of community members as providers of health services to fellow members of the community (as health educators/promoters, community counsellors, family planning or primary health care workers, and health volunteers) is a common type of community participation. Their services may be provided in the individual household, in the broader community context, or in a facility (static or mobile).

Another type of community participation is centred on the assumption of individual responsibility for one's own health. In order for health status at the community level to be improved, not only must individuals have essential health knowledge and take responsibility for those actions which they can change within the parameters of their daily living conditions but, in addition, each must recognize the value of public health, preventive and curative services, know where such services are provided, when to use them and finally, utilize them appropriately. The importance of this type of personalized community participation should not be overlooked. Especially in urban communities which have higher levels of education, this form may appropriately be dominant.

Nothing precludes a community from simultaneously sustaining different types of participation, nor should one type of participation be viewed as superior to another. Which types of participation are the most appropriate for an urban community, and hence the easiest to mobilize, may depend on the inherent characteristics of that community, such as those presented in Box 2.2.

Identification and advocacy for linkages between systems and structures

Community based public health, family planning and primary health care (PHC) services cannot exist in isolation. If the services are to have their maximal effect through appropriate utilization, they must be linked

Box 2.1

TYPES OF URBAN COMMUNITY PARTICIPATION

Advocacy
Relaying the specific health needs/services of the urban community to decision or policy makers and authorities responsible for health related conditions or services; following the process to assume those needs/services are obtained.

Information sharing; awareness building
Serving as the informal or formal conduit for information regarding health services or health promotion/ education between members of the community.

Community liaison functions
Actions performed to 'link' members of urban households with health services needed or desired; participatory activities may range from simple transfer of information regarding location of facility/provider or hours of operation to actual accompaniment of the individual to the appropriate provider/facility; critical function in terms of increasing utilization of existing services/facilities.

Direct service provision
Performance of health promotion, preventive health education or curative health services, whether delivered in the household, community, outreach site or fixed facility; may be volunteer service or service provided through a formal position within the health delivery system.

Supervision of community health services (providers/facilities)
Active role in supervising the staff providing community health services (volunteers or paid workers/professionals) at the facility or system level.

Management of health services provided in/for the community
Role in decisions regarding planning, setting priorities for services, identification of candidates, recruitment/selection of providers (health liaison volunteers or paid professional health care staff), and allocation of resources for services – may be at facility level (eg for community based clinic) or at system level (eg for urban wardwide community volunteer network or municipal health outreach facilities).

Financial or material support
Community contribution of space, equipment or supplies, materials for facility construction or financial support/cost sharing for provision of community health services (eg salaries of providers, initial capital for facility or later operational costs of facility).

In-kind contribution
Labour for facility construction or maintenance, unpaid time devoted to the development and implementation/operation of urban community health and related services.

Self-help
Individual or household level actions taken to improve health status of members, including increasing knowledge regarding habits and practices which promote health, as well as adoption of behaviours or participation in activities which maintain or improve the health of the household/family members.

Box 2.2

CHARACTERISTICS WHICH INFLUENCE TYPE AND LEVEL OF COMMUNITY PARTICIPATION IN URBAN HEALTH

Geography and demographics
- Spatial configuration and geography
- Population size and density
- Growth rate and pattern (natural increase, migration) of community
- Degree of mobility of community
- Gender and age profiles of community; dominant/majority groups
- Educational levels of community; degree of literacy or non-literacy

Economy
- Economic base: manufacturing, agriculture, service etc
- Size, economic importance of informal sector
- Prosperity level: percentage living in poverty; degree of inequality of income

Sociocultural
- Most prevalent family structure
- Duration of urban residence/community-specific residence
- Frequency of neighbour contacts/usual mode of social contact
- Mobility of women
- Dominant community ideologies
- Strength of community links with rural 'home' village and traditions

Organizational capacity
- Strength of community identity
- Type of community: geographic, common tradition/value or cause, epidemiologic risk
- History of crisis/cause which effectively mobilized community action (springboard)
- Existing community organizational structures (formal or informal)
- Presence of strong, recognized local leader(s)
- Recognized consensus regarding health or health services priority issue

Health status and delivery system
- Administrative structure for services
- Status of physical service needs
- Status of social service needs

Government role and responsibilities/inputs
- Level of government involvement/provision of health services; government Ministry responsible for urban health
- Current government policy regarding urban/municipal health services; equity of services
- Level of government resources available/allocated for health services

Private sector strength
- Level of nongovernmental services and resources for health services

Source: partly adapted from McGee and Young (1986)

at one end with households at risk, and at the other with secondary health care facilities or other health related services. Unfortunately, there is growing evidence that urban dwellers, despite geographic proximity, may not utilize existing health services (for example unimmunized children living within view of an EPI outreach or fixed site; children dying from dehydration within walking distance of a referral and treatment hospital) (Bulut et al 1991, Baqui et al 1993, Lastonet et al 1993). Thus, linkages between branches of urban health systems (family planning and PHC) are important, as are those between the health system and other sectors which provide services that influence health status. In addition, formalized, effective mechanisms for referral between the different levels or tiers of the health delivery system (ie community based and secondary and tertiary facilities); as well as between public sector divisions (ie municipal and state, provincial, national); and between various health sectors (ie municipal and NGO) are critical to assure the provision of maximally effective urban primary health services. Intersystemic and multisectoral linkages are essential for optimal management, mobilization and use of the multiplicity of urban health resources available to a community.

Hence, perhaps one of the most important roles of the community is to identify and advocate for effective linkages between households and local health care extenders or outreach workers of preventive or curative primary health services (from the formal or informal health care delivery systems); or in those cases where no outreach tier exists, to facilitate connections with the fixed site primary health care or family planning facility which is delivering services (often in geographic proximity) to the community (however it is defined).

Advocacy for the development of intersectoral mechanisms for coordinated urban health planning is another important type of community participation. Within a typical city, the responsibilities for safe water, sanitation (solid waste disposal, garbage collection), transport systems and roads, urban housing and development, job skill-building, social welfare, health and hospitals lie within different departments or agencies. There is seldom a vehicle for these departments to work together in a coordinated fashion with an urban community to develop a plan of action which delegates responsibilities for activities to improve health services, promote individual health, or even to alleviate community poverty. Nonetheless, without such a framework for coordinated planning and implementation of activities, it is impossible for a community to collectively or individually 'activate' the necessary intersectoral institutions.

That is why it is so important for community members to have a clear understanding of their urban borders as related to the provision of urban services, to know the appropriate authorities and corresponding implementing agencies for various public services, as well as to know the names and titles of individuals in charge of each service for their community. It is a community responsibility to develop a repository of knowledge about agencies providing health and related public services, and to advocate the creation of an institutional framework between those agencies, which it can use to communicate needs and plans which address those needs. Therefore, urban communities can play an important role as health advocates and 'instigators' mobilizing the delivery of services to their members. But, this role must be learned; it is seldom a spontaneous development.

Another significant community role may be the identification of a critical mass of individuals who function as community health liaison persons, assuring linkage between households and the first available level of care in the health delivery system. Such an urban health liaison person should be a trusted member of the community and have the knowledge base to facilitate such linkage. The liaison function may be formally organized as part of the health delivery system, such as when included in the role of urban health volunteers (extenders of the formal health delivery system), or may be an ad hoc function outside of the health system, performed by respected elderly traditional leaders or those with higher education or experience who are not in the matrix of health system providers. In the latter case, the urban health liaison person may refer patients or clients to the urban community health volunteer.

Linkage between PHC services and those delivered at secondary or tertiary care facilities is also necessary, but should be the responsibility of the formal health care delivery system and not of the community.

Finally, the issue of urban poverty must at least be mentioned because of its untoward influence on the overall health of urban communities. Clearly, intersectoral, multi-agency approaches to mobilize community participation and resources are essential in the fight against urban poverty. Although the topic goes beyond the scope of this chapter, development of multiparty responsibility and participation (community and formal service agency) in the delivery of community based health services is a critical step in creating alliances and partnerships which can also be used to address urban poverty.

Mobilizing community leadership: examining urban obstacles to health and developing community solutions

Obviously there are many obstacles to health for urban dwellers which have been amply described in the literature and experienced by those trying to mobilize urban communities in the delivery of health services and the improvement of their health status. Some of the more common obstacles in the development of effective urban community-based health delivery systems include: mobility of individuals and households; heterogeneous populations; lack of familial support and disintegration of household social structure; poverty; non-literacy and low education; substance abuse, violence and crime; limited time; non-legal status of some urban dwellers; lack of political knowledge and will; intersectoral turf wars; and no clear lines of authority and responsibility between public sector agencies providing support.

In fact, although many of these attributes are functional obstacles to the delivery of health services and/or the mobilization of urban community participation in health care, some of them can be used to the advantage of an urban community. For example, changing sociocultural norms, the breakdown of traditional rural support networks and intergenerational familial ties can all constitute obstacles to health, but viewed from another perspective, may allow freedom from social constrictions which fosters new opportunities for women, ethnic groups and disadvantaged minorities. Urban women, especially those living in poverty, have been found to be open to new ideas which, in conjunction with increased social freedom, results in increased acceptance of preventive health practices such as immunizations or family planning (Jancloes et al 1985).

The critical roles and responsibilities which women and less educated members of the urban community play as urban health volunteers will be discussed further in the chapter, but often it is only in less restricted, poor urban environments that such roles blossom. Furthermore, changing norms often bring new opportunities for education and possibilities for employment, which ultimately results in better economic conditions and associated improvements in nutrition, housing or other essential determinants of health.

Likewise, the diversity and heterogeneity of cities makes the delivery of services more difficult, since the needs of subgroups may be quite variable, as are the modes of communication most effective to reach them. However, the inevitable exposure to a diversity of ideas and walks of life which urban heterogeneity spontaneously produces (although at times painfully), may also serve to 'open the eyes and minds', particularly of the less advantaged, to new achievements and life possibilities which they would seldom have experienced in more homogeneous rural environments.

Similarly, urban population density and crowding, which promote the transmission of communicable diseases, can be viewed simultaneously as 'allies' supportive of efficient and rapid delivery of services to large numbers of people.

Thus, an important next step in mobilizing urban community participation and that of their leaders is the identification of obstacles to the delivery and utilization of health services at the community level, followed by a careful examination of how such obstacles can be used to advantage, or at least addressed by appropriate solutions. Activities can then be developed to implement the agreed upon solutions or to develop them.

The most abundant resource in cities is the human resource! This is especially true in urban disadvantaged communities where untapped human potential abounds. Many individuals living in urban poverty possess immense inherent resources for survival; they are a repository of unique ideas for solutions to improve their own health within the realistic constraints of their environment. These individuals and their knowledge base must be incorporated into community solutions for the effective delivery of urban health services. They are often highly motivated, but may require the attention of an outside 'vehicle' to stimulate their participation (Jandoes et al 1985).

VEHICLES FOR MOBILIZING URBAN COMMUNITY PARTICIPATION AND DELIVERING COMMUNITY BASED PRIMARY HEALTH SERVICES

Those urban communities most in need of primary health services are the high risk, socioeconomically deprived communities. Precisely because of their poverty and consequent 'survival edge' mentality, as well as the attendant factors of low education, non-literacy, unemployment and a lack of familiarity with the power structure in a city, these communities often have great difficulty in organizing, much less mobilizing resources for their health needs. They are the 'silent majority' of the urban 'fourth world'. For these reasons, it is important to identify existing organizations such as the Municipal Department of Health (MDOH), urban medical schools or departments of community health, NGOs and international or donor organizations which can be used as 'vehicles' – to harness their expertise, energies and resources to develop partnerships with each other and with urban communities in need, to mobilize these communities and develop effective community-based primary health services. Several examples of each type of vehicle are described, from cities in Asia, Africa, and Latin America and the Caribbean. Mechanisms employed to establish a relationship with the community and ultimately to mobilize participation are summarized, as well as lessons or recommendations.

Municipal health departments

The responsibilities and resources of municipal departments of health vary greatly. However, increasingly with 'decentralization' becoming a common government objective, more authority and resources are shifting to local governments such as municipalities, both for health and other services. In many cases, the municipal government may not have the human resources or the administrative capacity to effectively assume this increased burden, but these realities are seldom considered in the decision to decentralize. Hence, decentralization poses a challenge to municipalities which deserves attention, a challenge which has particular importance for urban health.

Urban communities must develop a clear understanding of precisely the responsibilities and resources at the disposal of their municipal departments of health. Box 2.3 delineates important steps for the municipal government and subsequently its citizens to take in order to clarify roles, identify service responsibilities and capabilities as well as obvious gaps or duplication in regard to urban health.

It is important to analyze which public sector entity has the decision making authority; which has the implementational responsibility; and which has the budgetary or fiscal authority for health and related services. Suffice it to say, it may be quite difficult to obtain this information, especially as the dictates of decentralized policy may be legislated before corresponding implementation implications have been fully considered.

In some circumstances, especially when resources are limited, there may be unwritten 'agreements' between public sector agencies which transfer functional responsibility from one to the other, despite legislative responsibility on record. This has often been the case in cities: district or provincial Ministries of Health have concentrated on the non-urban communities under their jurisdiction, leaving the urban municipal communities to the Municipal Departments of Health, within the Municipal Local Government Authority.

Box 2.3

ESSENTIAL STEPS FOR RAPID IDENTIFICATION OF MUNICIPAL HEALTH SERVICES PER COMMUNITY (COVERAGE, GAPS OR DUPLICATION)

1 Identify the geographic or other 'functional borders' of the community.
2 Identify the specific responsibilities of the MDOH to provide health services for the constituents living in the community or services directly influencing the health status of its constituents – be clear as to the precise language which mandates these responsibilities.
3 Determine the number and location of municipal health facilities serving the community (all levels – community posts, PHC clinics or vaccination facilities, multipurpose clinics, hospitals) and the number/type of health positions allocated or sanctioned (as well as actually filled – for there is often a large discrepancy between the two).
4 Determine the number and location of health facilities and staff positions provided by the district or provincial health department within the Ministry of Health to serve the community.
5 Identify those health services and related facilities or staff most directly serving the community level and whether they are under the direction of the municipal or district/provincial government.
6 Identify other sectoral services which directly influence the health status of the community and which organization or division is directly responsible for them.
7 Map the sites of above noted municipal and district/provincial facilities for health services in relation to the target community.

Seldom are there coordinated efforts between the local government bodies and the district or provincial Ministry of Health to maximize use of their combined resources to assure effective, accessible urban health services for their communities. The development of urban health profiles, such as discussed below in regard to the Bangladesh Urban Immunization Project, in conjunction with mapping all available public and private health resources creates a fundamental fact sheet which can be used for coordinated planning.

One valuable role for urban communities is to bring their community health problems to the attention of the newly responsible municipal authorities. Again, mapping can be a valuable tool to rapidly identify communities without facilities, or to reveal obstacles to access which may not be known to those not residing in the area. As democratic practices gain momentum across the globe, municipal authorities will be increasingly sensitive to the needs of their electorates, granting communities an opportunity to champion health needs and bringing urban primary health care to the top of the political agenda (as we are now witnessing in the USA with health reform). Armed with this information, a community can decide whether or not it is important to forge a formal organizational link with the MDOH to mobilize the delivery of better community-based health services. Three different examples of MDOH mobilization are outlined below in Boxes 2.4, 2.5 and 2.6: Nairobi, Kampala, Dhaka.

Box 2.4

NAIROBI, KENYA

Key partners: Ministry of Local Government (Nairobi City Commission, Department of Public Health), Ministry of Health and National Council on Population and Development (NCPD) and African Medical Research Fund (AMREF)

General description: Three distinctive activities in Nairobi illustrate public-private sector partnerships as vehicles to stimulate and sustain urban community-based primary health care: the development of an urban Primary Health Care Unit in the Department of Public Health within the Nairobi City Council; a pilot project (Population, Environment, and Health/FP Services in Urban Slums) implemented by the City Council; and AMREF's Urban Child Survival Project. These activities have disparate funding and implementing mechanisms, but each has developed collaboratively.

Mechanisms used by NCC (MDOH) to establish relationship with and mobilize target urban community:

- Local administrative chiefs involved in early planning and to arrange initial community presentation
- Conducted slum community SES and demographic survey, sharing results with community leaders and field workers to increase awareness of problems and related objectives of project
- Developed collaborative committee to share information regarding services delivered by NGOs and Government of Kenya (GOK) in target communities
- Resource identification and mapping; identified all community-based health and family planning distributors (CBDs); held meeting of all CBDs to discuss operational issues such as selection criteria, services and catchment etc
- Encouraged community participation in rapid environmental assessment; presentation of results to community members and joint development of action plan with community participation
- Developed and trained slum health committees to oversee activities, under direction of local government chairman
- Project staff obtained mass media coverage and high level political support (Mayor) for launching of project at community level

Lessons learned:

- Communities often have internal capabilities to identify solutions for problems, but require initial guidance/information to start the problem solving process (initial organization, management and resource mobilization)
- Poor communities do recognize the benefit of communal activities and are willing to support such
- Members of slum communities are often willing to share the little they have, in contrast to their better off counterparts
- NGOs may be better accepted in slum communities, where suspicions of government may exist; new immigrants or non-legal squatters are particularly fearful of government and may resist services that require registration (immunizations, vital statistics at birth or death)
- Professional health workers from outside the slums may be unwilling or find it difficult to provide services in this environment

- More time is needed to establish urban community-based PHC services than rural ones, in part due to the heterogeneity and mobility of urban communities
- When a precedent of free externally provided services (public sector or NGO) has been established, the development of responsible community participation is more difficult
- Balancing the tensions or demands between project objectives/outputs required for funding and the community's desires/needs is an ongoing challenge for field staff
- Working/service hours of staff are/should be largely dictated by community needs
- Municipal expansion should be preceded by the development of health services for the new areas

Sources: Programme description (1993) J W Kinaro; (1993) Nairobi City Convention; (1993) Nairobi City Council's report on establishment of PHC units

Medical schools

It is common for medical schools and associated schools of public health or departments of community health to be located in urban settings. These can become powerful allies and supporters for the development of community based primary health care services. Not only do these institutions have human resources to assist in the delivery of services, but they also possess research capabilities which can be marshalled to identify and develop alternative solutions to health problems, including more efficient and effective modes of service delivery to high risk urban populations. In addition, medical schools produce the health providers of the future; if they can be sensitized to the importance of primary health care and the urgent needs of urban communities in this regard, larger numbers may devote their professional energies to this neglected area, including direct employment in the urban public or private sectors focused on services for the urban poor.

Medical school partnership with municipal departments of health may take many forms including:

- direct secondment of faculty to the MDOH for a period of time (which affords a real world experience for faculty who are normally removed from politics and the municipal administrative bureaucracies);
- student interns who rotate through the MDOH and assist as requested on assignments (again providing important exposure to realistic situations and an alternative use of their medical degrees not usually afforded in the standard curricula);
- development of a collaborative project effort focused on a particular community (providing the city with additional human resources and the medical school with a field site for teaching the principles of community primary health care);
- development of a curriculum which includes long term work in a community, labour and technical assistance supported by the medical school but with the administrative and logistical support of the MDOH (extension of the MDOH services at minimal cost and

Box 2.5

KAMPALA, UGANDA

Key partners: Government of Uganda, Ministry of Finance (GOU/MOF), Kampala City Council (KCC) – Department of Public Health and Labour Intensive Work Unit (local government) and UNDP.

General description: A drainage repair project in Kampala City was used as an entry point for PHC and community mobilization in an urban slum

History: In the 1950s, the municipality built a drainage system of temporary materials which had not been maintained; in 1992, UNDP (through the Ministry of Finance) agreed to finance reconstruction of this drain with permanent materials; Kampala City Council (KCC) Medical Officer saw the opportunity to use the project as an entry point for PHC in slums through which the pipe ran and successfully convinced the GOU/MOF, UNDP and KCC to add a community-based PHC component to the project.

Mechanisms used by KCC (MDOH) to establish relationship with and mobilize target urban community:
Community seminars and meetings, facilitated by representatives of different organizations or government sectors (Ministry of Health, Ministry of Agriculture, Institute of Public Health, local university, hospitals, NGOs, and KCC's Town Planning and Development Unit)
- Conducted community meetings initially with zonal chairmen and secretaries to explain project and select representatives for a project committee
- Held series of community seminars and films on health topics for residents identified in community survey; community invited to discuss participatory solutions and behavioural changes needed
- Focused some community seminars on perceived community needs in health services, but also examined obstacles to meeting those needs, as well as identified local resources to assist and implement services
- Conducted community training on selected income generating projects (IGP)

Lessons learned:
- It takes time to develop trust between the local community and government authority
- Slum dwellers may harbour mistrust of collaborative efforts due to past experiences with broken promises ('briefcase' NGOs)
- Lack of land tenure is an underlying issue; since tenancy is not secure, some community members ask Why waste effort on improving sites?

Recommendations:
- Use health and SES survey information to mobilize community and obtain agreement on priority joint actions as well as solutions
- Include landlords in mobilization and health education; encourage their participation and support for structural improvements
- Ongoing remuneration for committee member time is needed for sustainability; this is one role of the city corporation

Unique contribution: intersectoral collaboration; use of engineering infrastructural improvement as entree for community PHC (collaboration of engineers and health within City Government)

Source: (1994) Programme description J R M Wayira

Box 2.6

DHAKA, BANGLADESH

Key partners: Government of Bangladesh (GOB) – Ministry of Local Government, Rural Development and Cooperatives (MOLGRDC), Ministry of Health and Family Welfare (MOHFW) and USAID (international donor)

History: In the late 1980s, it was recognized that urban immunization rates in Bangladesh lagged considerably behind rural rates, and the national immunization plan had been developed with rural programmes in mind, neglecting urban needs. USAID agreed to support strengthening of urban immunization services in 88 municipalities of Bangladesh (essentially all municipalities at that time, though number has since grown).

Mechanisms used by MOLGRDC to establish relationship with and mobilize target urban community:
• Established formal political commitment and collaboration between public sector agents: Ministry of Health and Family Welfare and Ministry of Local Government
• Performed baseline assessments of immunization coverage; used findings to advocate expanded support from municipal authorities for urban EPI services, especially for the urban poor
• Developed and implemented urban-specific EPI plans and activities
• Sponsored awareness-raising activities in conjunction with UNICEF eg signs, radio and TV programmes, press coverage, use of sports and entertainment figures; developed entertainment education video film for local use at community events
• Performed studies of urban slum communications to develop appropriate strategies to reach these populations
• Developed and implemented school lesson plans including EPI to teach as well as involve students in immunization promotion

Lessons learned:
• There is a need to develop local government capacity to perform local area planning for urban EPI services
• Inter-Ministerial collaboration is essential, a formal policy and mechanism to address division of roles, responsibilities, and to conduct ongoing joint planning is required
• Urban-specific IEC and communications strategies must be developed; emphasis on increasing knowledge of urban slum populations in order to create demand for immunization services is important

Recommendations:
• The MOLGRDC should be specifically included as an additional collaborative partner in immunizations along with the MOHFW (previous agreements with USAID focused on the MOHFW)
• The city corporations/municipalities will be the local implementing agencies for immunizations

Sources: (1994) Carnell M and Hossain K, Urban PHC Task Force Report; (1992) Favin M and EPI Directorate, Reports on Bangladesh's Urban EPI Project; (1994) Carnell M and Hossain K, Forging Intersectoral Partnerships for Urban Health in Bangladesh

indepth exposure to the complications and challenges of urban PHC for the medical school participants – faculty and students); and

- operational research projects developed within a curriculum or as independent projects which address specific issues noted by community and/or MDOH to be important deterrents to improved service delivery or the promotion of health in the cities (opportunity to define new solutions at minimal cost to community or the MDOH, but for which neither usually has internal resources (time or money) to address independently).

Medical schools may also develop independent activities and relationships with a community, or may work in conjunction with NGO partners – two examples of independent medical school initiatives are given in Boxes 2.7 and 2.8, as well as one example of a non-local university providing international support for an urban health project (Box 2.9).

Non–governmental organizations

There is often distrust of government, whether it be municipal or national, among the urban poor communities, those most in need of urban primary health care services. Part of this distrust stems from the 'non legal' status of some urban settlers, or the fact that the government may be comprised of individuals from a different ethnic, religious or tribal affiliation than the communities it serves; but the socio-economic and educational disparities between government employees and members of the urban underserved communities create a barrier in themselves. Finally, all too often these communities have suffered at the hands of government decisions to 'clean up' their living sites, which usually translated into overnight demolition, without replacement. Hence, it is often difficult for government, specifically the MDOH, to overcome such ingrained barriers and to effectively involve communities in decision making regarding their priority health needs or participation in health committees.

For these reasons, Non-governmental organizations (NGOs) or private voluntary organizations (PVOs) can often play a special role in reaching and mobilizing urban communities. When they team with the MDOH, NGOs can provide expertise and experience in community organization which many MDOHs do not possess, as well as augmenting the delivery of community-based PHC services. Furthermore, NGOs generally are quite successful at implementing small scale local projects, often with impressive improvements in the health status of those they serve; but they have been less adept in translating such successes into large scale applications, in part because they do not create the original project within the context of a replicable unit or framework. Thus, a partnership between MDOHs and NGOs provides the NGO with a macro perspective and a replicable unit of operation (ie the municipal ward or district); and the MDOH with a more trusting mode of entry into the community, as well as expertise in grassroots community organization and mobilization, and the means to deliver community-based primary health care services, with special emphasis on prevention (versus facility based curative care, more common to MDOH providers).

Box 2.7

AGA KHAN UNIVERSITY/MEDICAL SCHOOL – KARACHI, PAKISTAN

Aga Khan University, a private university in Pakistan, is an advocate for 'concerted interaction between community, government, and the health system (both public and private)' (Bryant 1991). The objectives of the Department of Community Health in the Medical School exemplify this belief: '1) strengthen the development of health systems in Pakistan through education and research, with emphasis on the development and implementation of health system prototypes in collaboration with local and national authorities; and 2) educate health personnel for leadership in dealing with health and development problems, particularly those of the more deprived communities...' (Bryant 1991).

The University's primary health care programme addressed the problems of extreme urban poverty coupled with inadequate government health services by focusing on the development of small community-based systems that were effective, affordable and amenable to replication. It established seven urban PHC models in Karachi, six in low income 'katchi abadis' (each serving a community of roughly 10, 000 inhabitants), and one in a lower middle income area. Within these settings, the University used different methods to initiate and develop community-based urban PHC: university-led, community-led and joint health promotion/disease prevention.

Five of the models followed the *university-led* approach. In these models, there were three tiers of health personnel: community-based health workers recruited from the target community and trained in the community to provide local services; paramedical lady health visitors who provided supervision and support for the community-based workers; and a community health nurse and/or doctor who supervised the lady health visitors. Most service was provided by the community-based workers, each covering about 125 households with preventive services (immunizations, growth monitoring), oral rehydration therapy, recognition and referral of acute respiratory infections, and identification and referral of high risk pregnancies.

Community participation (outside of community health workers) was usually concentrated in health related supportive activities such as income generation, health education, and advocacy for clean water and sanitation. The health data collected by CHWs was used by the health professionals in the system, but the community was not involved in the collection or use of such data.

The *community-led* model was supported through a local NGO which encouraged and motivated community members to learn about the causes of ill health and to identify their own solutions. Decision making was shared between the community organization and the university providers, but otherwise the three tiers of the delivery system were the same as the university model. It took considerably longer to establish this model.

The *health promotion/prevention* model was instituted in the lower middle income area and utilized community volunteers as well as private medical practitioners to identify risk groups, improve health awareness attitudes and practices, and treat/refer as necessary.

In general, the university-led models were able to demonstrate significant improvements in coverage and impact indicators in a shorter time, in contrast to the community-led programme which required more time to develop, and consequently showed less improvement in those health indicators monitored. However, it appears as though the latter has sustained a larger and more vibrant community involvement than the university-led programmes.

Source: (1993) Bryant J, Marsh D and Khan K et al, A Developing Country's University Oriented Toward Strengthening Health Systems *Am Journal Public Health* pp1537–1543, (1991) Bryant, J 'The role of third world universities in health development' *Asia Pacific Journal of Public Health*

Box 2.8

UNIVERSITY OF ST ROSARIO – BOGOTÁ, COLOMBIA

The Community Health Programme in the School of Medicine supervises the provision of services by students participating in its community-based model located in an urban marginal 'barrio' neighbourhood. Its programme is constructed around didactics and experiential learning based on four modules, which together promote 'health for all and sustainable development':

- community participation;
- preventive and curative ambulatory care services;
- administration; and
- medical education.

Medical students as well as other health related professionals in training take part in the community-based maternal and child health services, oral health services, mental health services and adolescent school health programme. Forty medical students per semester take part in the programme, each providing care to approximately 14 families. The students not only gain experience in providing community-based healthcare services, but also are taught through experience to evaluate those services, to perform community-based health status surveys and use such data in the development and monitoring of health programmes, and to organize/facilitate community organization.

The Community Health Programme has established working collaborations with other government institutions and with NGOs in the area. The Medical School thus becomes a vehicle for improving essential community-based services for an underserved barrio population, while simultaneously developing the capacities of future community health providers.

Source: (1993) Latorre, C *Programme Description*

Box 2.9

JOHNS HOPKINS UNIVERSITY/ICDDR,B – DHAKA, BANGLADESH

Johns Hopkins University (JHU), School of Hygiene and Public Health, Department of International Health provides technical assistance to the Urban Health Extension Project of the International Centre for Diarrhoeal Disease Research, Bangladesh (ICDDR,B). ICDDR,B is an autonomous, nonprofit organization performing research, and providing education, training and clinical services. The Centre's mandate is to undertake and promote research on diarrhoeal diseases, and related subjects of acute respiratory infections, nutrition and fertility with the aim of preventing and controlling diarrhoeal diseases and improving health care.

The Urban Health Extension Project (UHEP), formerly the Urban Volunteer Programme (UVP), was conceived as an operations research project to test the feasibility, effectiveness and impact of a volunteer extender health delivery system, using female volunteers – women from slum communities – to provide preventive healthcare and referral services to their fellow residents in Dhaka. Originally, the focus of the programme was on diarrhoeal disease prevention and management through health education and the distribution of oral rehydration solution (ORS) packets, but the services were extended to include immunization, nutrition education and Vitamin A capsule distribution, and family planning. The target population of the project was children under five years (and their caretakers/mothers) living in the urban slums of Dhaka.

Collaborating institutions: Government of Bangladesh – MOHFW and MOLGDRC; Dhaka City Corporation; ICDDR,B; JHU; local NGO – Concerned Women for Family Planning

The UVP/UHEP/UORP has served to stimulate multi-agency support for an innovative health surveillance system documenting the health status of urban poor children, as well as promoting the need for urban community-based FP-MCH and child health services. Its work has resulted in a new and more robust collaboration between public sectors – Ministry of Health and Family Welfare, Directorates of Health and Family Planning, with the MOLGRDC; private sector (NGO), as well as renewed partnership with JHU and ICDDR,B. These latter institutions served as vehicles to raise awareness of the plight of the urban poor and the need to develop urban health interventions and community-based delivery systems, using local capacities and participation.

While performing operations research and developing urban health delivery system models, the projects also provided much needed services to urban slum mothers and their children. The community-based volunteer extension delivery system linked slum dwellers with primary health care providers. With growing knowledge and maturity of the research, formal mechanisms to transfer capabilities and apply systems within existing public and private sector frameworks are being developed. The process has taken over a decade; perhaps application of this experience will decrease the time needed elsewhere. Such successful mating of research institutions with community and government health systems merits close examination for application in other cities.

Sources: (1993) ICDDR, B, *Working papers nos 32, 33 and 36*

Furthermore, it is not uncommon for NGOs (for the purposes of this discussion, religious organizations such as missions can be included in this group) to target their services to underserved, less privileged communities. Therefore, in some instances, NGOs choose to develop their own independent relations with communities from which they mobilize and launch community health projects. However, as more NGOs rely on international agencies or bilateral donor support, their projects have come under increased scrutiny – particularly in regard to sustainability and replicability, or implementation on a larger scale. Thus, in more recent years, several NGO–MDOH partnerships have been initiated. And, in other cases, even when there has not been a partnership, close communications and dissemination of experience has assured the transferral of vital information to the MDOH. While further discussion of NGOs can be found in the chapter by Atkinson, Box 2.10 presents a case study from Bangladesh which demonstrates collaboration between an MDOH and an NGO. Another example of an NGO vehicle, AMREF in Nairobi, was described under the MDOH section.

International organizations and international donor development and aid agencies

'International organizations' refers largely to UN bodies such as UNDP, UNICEF, WHO, or the World Bank (sometimes called multilaterals). International donor development and aid agencies (sometimes called bilaterals) include those agencies responsible for the oversight and implementation of a country's development activities such as GTZ, ODA, USAID, DANIDA. These organizations do not act independently in any country, and most commonly have formal agreements with the presiding national government. In most cases, their support for health interventions and services is channelled through the Ministry of Health. However, as awareness grows regarding the appalling health status and attendant inadequate services for the urban poor, several organizations have developed relationships and support to MDOHs/MOLG, providing a new partnership model worthy of consideration. Further details about international organizations' support for urban health can be found in the chapters by Goldstein et al, Hecht, Padmini, Fluty and Lissfelt, and Merkle and Knobloch.

Two examples follow in Boxes 2.11 and 2.12. The first is directed at improving an urban hospital's ability to serve its catchment communities and is an example of MDOH-international development agency collaboration; the second, with an objective to 'build the capacity of city and municipal governments to implement cost-effective slum health and nutrition programmes, in partnership with communities' represents a partnership between an international organization (World Bank) and the MDOH. A third example which focused on a particular child health intervention (EPI) and involved an international development agency has already been discussed under the section regarding MDOH.

Box 2.10

WORLD VISION – DHAKA, BANGLADESH

Key partner: Dhaka City Corporation (MOLGRDC)

General description: World Vision began its urban slum project in Dhaka in 1988 to educate and motivate poor families to adopt selective 'child protective' health behaviours: family planning; immunizations for mothers and children; breastfeeding; weaning food practices; use of ORS during diarrhoea; Vitamin A supplementation; and referral for treatment of illness. Community outreach and support for maintaining these improved health practices was instituted through a grassroots level system of Neighbourhood Health Committees (NHC), Community Volunteers (CVs) and Focus Mother Groups (FMG). The catchment population of the project, one 'ward', was based on Dhaka's municipal administrative system. The average population of a ward in Dhaka is 50,000–100,000 inhabitants – the project ward was estimated to have a population of 77,000. At the start of the Project, there was no local infrastructure easily identified in terms of local leaders or organizations; no maps, local level health, demographic or socioeconomic data; and no reliable household identification system.

Mechanisms used to establish relationship with and mobilize target urban community:
- Development of grassroots infrastructure within overall superstructure of City Corporation's administrative system, using the 'ward' as local replication unit
- Use of local crisis (flood) to mobilize participation/responsibility of community local leaders, as well as to instill a recognition of the importance of health and sanitation in all residents

Lessons learned:
- Establishing pilot projects within a functional municipal administrative infrastructure increases the likelihood of replicability and expansion, as does involving municipal or city local government authorities in the design and implementation of the project
- Mapping of focused local areas by community members is a powerful tool to foster community awareness, stimulate participation, and promote resource identification
- Most urban families, even poor ones, are willing and able to pay at least a minimal fee for services
- The inclusion of all socio-economic groups in a project design and implementation may improve its chance of financial sustainability

Recommendations:
- Strengthen local government and infrastructure capabilities in health management skills, community organizing, planning and resource identification
- Integrated health/development urban plans should be developed for cities/municipalities which clearly identify the contributions and roles of public and private sectors
- Communities as well as local government and Ministry of Health need to be involved in the design of urban health projects; most donor agencies do not allow time to develop participation in project design, but such is critical for sustainability of community support

Source: (1991) *Kamalapur Child Survival Project, Final Evaluation Report*

Box 2.11

GERMAN GOVERNMENT/GTZ – LOMÉ, TOGO

GTZ's experience in Lomé illustrates that 'urban community participation may be better understood if it is considered as a progressive, evolving process over time; and expressed as a collaboration between the community and the local health professionals' (Schmidt-Ehry Gertrud 1993). Between 1988 and 1993, the German Government financed a Mother and Child Health Care Project in Lomé, Togo. GTZ was the executing agency for the project which developed out of the need to create a new maternity facility to relieve the congestion and overload at the University Clinic.

It was decided that the existing health centre which offered outpatient services and MCH care could be expanded to include maternity labour and delivery/basic obstetric services. However, even after expansion and the addition of inpatient maternity services, it continued to function as a first contact primary health care facility for many of its constituents, primarily because there were no other affordable community-based primary health care facilities available. After several years of organizational transformations, the Health Centre was formally christened a Secondary Hospital in 1992. The Unit Heads of the hospital, along with several additional employees became responsible for planning, evaluation and operations of the Hospital.

Originally, the health system assessment of community needs and the subsequent planning was performed by health professionals using standard service utilization and demographic data; there was no input from community members, nor was there a mechanism to obtain such. With the construction of the maternity unit extension, GTZ encouraged involvement of the client community to better delineate their perceived service needs. Consequently, a health committee was established with the assistance of the Development Committee of the community. (This latter Committee was founded by the community itself in the 1980s to identify and contact NGOs that might help with financing projects addressing locally identified needs of unemployment, lack of sanitation and insufficient local health services.)

Lessons learned:
- Even though a rererral hospital is not the traditional nidus for community participation, in urban settings which frequently lack community based primary health care systems, a hospital can serve as a vehicle to mobilize community participation through the establishment of a representative health committee.
- Community health committee members need management and financial training to assure capable, meaningful participation.
- The composition, qualifications and skills needed, as well as the range of responsibilities/tasks of the community health committee will change over time.
- Political and legal authority for health management decisions may become more onerous in the future, making community participation less likely or feasible.
- Urban community heterogeneity makes initial representation dlfficult.
- Trust, confidence, and mutual respect between community members and health professionals must be established if community health committees are to be effective.

- Health committees should be open to recognizing nonhealth priority concerns of the community and facilitating intersectoral collaborations to address such issues.
- The most successful community participation occurred through smaller, organized pre-existing community groups which served as collaborative partners, facilitating cornmunity-health professional interactions; thus, such smaller community groups can serve as the voice of the larger community.
- Flexibility and rapid response to identified problems builds community confidence and trust, ultimately fueling participation.

Source: (1993) Schmidt-Ehry; G *Community Participation in an Urban Context* GTZ, Germany

---

Box 2.12

WORLD BANK – MANILA, PHILIPPINES

A major commitment by the World Bank and the Government of the Philippines Ministry of Health has been made to address urban poverty alleviation through improving the health and nutritional status of slum dwellers in three metropolitan areas. The project proposes to extend basic health and nutrition services to more than six million slum dwellers; to improve the quality of those services; and to stimulate community demand for services. Although this project is in the early stages of implementation, the planning, political commitment, policy development and information collected prior to its formal initiation, merit examination for their intrinsic value promoting and facilitating the role of urban communities (in addition to their necessary contribution to ultimate project implementation). The timeframe of the project is 1994–1998.

Strategies include:
- increasing resource flows for primary health and nutrition services in the slums and the ability to target these resources more tightly on those in need;
- using training, technical assistance and financial support to strengthen local government capabilities to manage improved health and nutrition services;
- building on experiences of the Philippines Health Department and UNICEF'S Urban Basic Services Programme to mobilize communities through partnerships with local government units and NGOs.

This project may be one of the largest and most significant commitments made to improving the health of the urban poor. It is also important because of its dedication to assisting the DOH to identify and fulfill its new role after devolution (providing support and guidelines rather than direct management of the health departments of local governments). Lessons can be applied in other urban environments where the impact and implications of decentralization policies are just coming to the fore. Another important contribution of the project is the development of tools and instruments to target services and resources to high risk urban populations such as in the slums. Ocular surveys were performed covering 40 per cent of the target cities to identify the geographical location of slums, estimated populations and type of slum settlement. A computerized urban geographic and health information system as well as an environmental assessment system have been developed which should be extremely valuable for health planning and monitoring.

Critical urban and slum policy decisions include the legalization of the delivery of health services to slums, regardless of land tenure status, and the development of a new health region covering the national capital region known as 'metro Manila' to strengthen public health and city services and to allow additional international aid, as well as technical and financial resources, to be channelled to the needy municipal health departments.

Source: (1993) Ureta, F *Urban Health and Nutrition Project, Philippines* World Bank

REFERENCES

Baquis, A, Paligor, N, Silimperi, D (!993) 'The prevention and treatment of diarrhoea in Dhaka slums' ICDDR B working paper no 32

Bulut, A Uzel, N Kutluay, T and Neyzi, O (1991) Experiences of a Health Team Working in a New Urban Settlement Area in Istanbul *Journal of Community Health* Human Science Press, Inc, Turkey, 16, pp251–258

Hughart, N Silimperi, D and Khatun, J (1992) A New EPI Strategy to Reach High Risk Urban Children in Bangladesh: Urban Volunteers *Journal of Tropical and Geographic Medicine* (1–2), pp144–148

Jancloes, M Seck, B van De Velden, L and Ndiaye, B (1985) Financing Urban Primary Health Services *Tropical Doctor*, pp98–104

Laston, S L, Baqui, A H, Paljor, N, Silimperi, D (1993) 'Immunization beliefs and coverage in Dhaka urban slums' ICDDR, B working paper no 33

Loewy, E (1987) Communities, Obligations, and Health Care *Social Science and Medicine*, 25, pp783–791

Management Sciences for Health, FPMD (1992) *The Family Planning Manager.* Using Maps to Improve Services vol 1 no 5.

McGee, T and Yeung, Y (1986) Participatory Urban Services in Asia *Community Participation in Delivering Urban Services in Asia* International Development Research Centre, Canada

Rakowski, C and Kastner, G (1985) Difficulties Involved in Taking Health Services to the People *Social Science and Medicine*, 21, pp67–75

Rifkin, S (1987) Primary Health Care, Community Participation and the Urban Poor: a Review of the Problems and Solution *Asia-Pacific Journal of Public Health* 1, pp57–63

Rifkin, S, Muller, I, Bichmann, W (1988) Primary health care: On measuring participation *Social Science and Medicine* 26 (9): 931–940

Rossi-Espagnet, A (1983) Primary Health Care in the Context of Rapid Urbanization *Community Development Journal*, 18, pp104–119

Silimperi, D (1994) *Delivering Child Survival Services to High Risk Population (Draft),* BASICS Strategy Paper, pp1–57

3

Features and Determinants of Urban Health Status

Marcel Tanner and Trudy Harpham (eds)

INTRODUCTION

Urbanization in the southern hemisphere is rapidly increasing, and estimates indicate that more than half of the global population will live in urban agglomerations in the next century (WHO 1992, World Bank 1992). The consequences for the health status of these urban and peri-urban populations are substantial and call for comprehensive attention and public health action. The health problems which are typical for the South, such as infectious diseases like measles, meningitis, malaria, cholera and AIDS, will remain and even increase. In addition, many health problems associated with the developed world, which until now have occurred predominantly in the North – such as cardiovascular disease and chronic diseases like diabetes and cancer – will substantially increase (Jamison et al 1993). The plethora of social problems linked to urbanization (Harpham et al 1988, Rossi-Espagnet et al 1991) have led and will continue to lead to important psychosocial problems, and are a key factor for the social development of the urban areas. Although the features of the epidemiological transition and the dimensions of the psychosocial problems have been described in detail (reviews in Harpham et al 1988, Jamison et al 1993), the determinants have so far not been well analyzed and understood. In particular, the effects of urbanization on health status, on the health behaviour of the population, and on the impact of health interventions are not well established. It is possible that a number of health problems which can be observed in cities in the South are not so much due to the urbanization process *per se* as to the overall changes in lifestyle which accompany urbanization.

Given this situation, urban health development can only be successful if it is integrated into the social and economic development approaches in a particular setting, and if it pursues the following specific objectives:

* Based on contributions by Maria Ducci, Peter Kilima, Ngudup Paljor, Voahangy Ramahatafandry and John Seager

- to improve health status;
- to achieve efficient use of resources with regard to allocation and utilization;
- to achieve equity with particular reference to access to and utilization of health care and promotion;
- to achieve consumer satisfaction by offering choices; and
- to look at costs, cost containment and cost control.

The present chapter summarizes the determinants of urban health status. Available data were reviewed and compared with rural data from the same country in order to reveal the distinct patterns of the health status of urban populations. Although the analysis considered an entire city, particular attention was paid to the poor, low income segments of the urban population. Therefore, we do not aim at a comprehensive review of all the available literature, but rather intend to illustrate major determinants, facts or trends with some representative, well-documented case studies.

IMPORTANT FEATURES OF HEALTH STATUS IN AN URBAN SETTING

Intra-urban differentials with regard to health status and demographic changes are considered to be the most crucial features for investigations of the underlying biomedical, sociocultural and economic determinants of health. A review of the available literature reveals a substantial lack of data on such differentials. Although we find comprehensive data sets for urban areas, based on routine health information systems or special surveys, real differences or unifying features are lost in most data sets as a consequence of the aggregation of data across wide social and economic groupings. Nevertheless, such information is crucial when one attempts to identify high risk groups or areas that require the attention of planners and subsequent public health action. A first step to fill this gap has been a large project on intra-urban health differentials in São Paulo and Accra, the results of which will soon be published (Stephens et al 1994).

Intra-urban differentials are a major feature of an analysis of urban health status and demand specific attention. The example in Table 3.1 illustrates this. It shows that the overall infant mortality rate (IMR) in Bangladesh appears more favourable for urban areas than for rural areas. However, once that data is disaggregated, the urban slums not only reach the highest IMR in the country but also show important gender differentials. An analysis of the available data shows that data on the changing patterns of morbidity and mortality that accompany the epidemiological transition in developing countries, and particularly on its effect in urban settings, are still very limited. There is a particularly acute lack of disaggregated data with regard to adult health in urban areas, and with regard to the occupational and environmental health risks and effects. It is therefore virtually impossible to assess the burden of disease faced by an urban population or a particular population stratum, following the concept of the World Development Report 1993 (World Bank 1993), in any city. This in turn renders rational priority setting and planning of health care delivery and promotion services very difficult.

Table 3.1 *Intra-urban differentials: infant mortality rate as an example –*
Bangladesh 1991 (1990)

	National[a]	Rural[b]	Urban[b]	Urban slums[c]
Total	**90 (94)**	**93 (97)**	**68 (71)**	**134**
Male	98 (98)	97 (101)	70 (73)	123
Female	91 (91)	89 (93)	65 (68)	146

Notes:
a) *Source:* Bangladesh Demographic Statistics, Bangladesh Bureau of Statistics,
Government of Bangladesh
b) *Source:* As a), but extrapolated from 1990 data (1991 Statistical Yearbook of Bangladesh)
c) *Source:* Urban Surveillance System, Urban Health Extension Project, ICDDR,B

Besides the intra-urban differentials, the comparison of the urban health
status with that of rural settings in the same country is of great
importance to understand the stage and process of the epidemiological
transition. The comparison of health status data between urban and rural
areas often reveals striking differences. Generally there is a higher risk of
dying from chronic, degenerative and cardiovascular diseases in urban
areas, whereas infectious diseases are leading causes of death in rural
areas. A similar situation is revealed for morbidity.

Table 3.2 *Selected causes of mortality by rural and urban areas – Mexico 1990*
(rates by 100,000 inhabitants)

Causes of mortality	Overall rate	Rural rate[a]	Urban rate[b]	Relative risk urban/ rural
Total	**520.37**	**530.68**	**516.23**	**0.97**
Heart Diseases	34.92	25.44	38.71	1.52
Diabetes Mellitus	31.73	17.02	37.64	2.21
Malignant Neoplasms	27.48	20.77	30.17	1.45
Pneumonia	26.86	34.39	23.84	0.69
Accidents	25.67	22.16	27.07	1.22
Diarrhoea and Gastroenteritis	23.67	40.41	16.95	0.42
Liver Diseases	23.03	19.94	22.87	1.15
Cerebrovascular Diseases	16.95	16.07	17.30	1.08
Certain Conditions Originating in the Perinatal Period	16.40	12.62	17.92	1.42
Malnutrition	14.00	19.78	11.68	0.59
Asthma	11.85	13.91	11.02	0.79
Nephropathy, Nephrotic and Nephritic Syndrome	10.18	8.48	10.86	1.28
Cardiac Arrhythmias	8.30	12.38	6.66	0.54
Chronic Lower Respiratory Diseases	6.75	4.42	7.69	1.74
Congenital Malformations	6.72	4.80	7.49	1.56

Table 3.2 (*continued*)

Causes of mortality	Overall rate	Rural rate	Urban rate	Relative risk urban/ rural
Tuberculosis	6.69	9.20	5.68	0.62
Other Anaemias	5.51	8.07	4.48	0.56
Peptic Ulcer	3.74	4.37	3.49	0.80
Septicaemia	3.48	2.97	3.68	1.24
Mental and Behavioural Disorders Due to Use of Alcohol	3.16	3.40	3.06	0.90
Acute Lower Respiratory Infections	2.16	3.43	1.65	0.48

Notes:
a) Places with ≤ 2500 inhabitants
b) Places with > 2500 inhabitants
Source: Special Printouts from Deaths Registration: Tape INEGI 1990

Table 3.3 *Prevalence and prevalence ratio of selected diseases by rural and urban places – Mexico 1987 (rates by 100,000 inhabitants)*

Selected diseases	Rural rate[a]	Urban rate[b]	Prevalence ratio urban/rural
Total	**60.40**	**48.10**	**0.80**
Diarrhoea	185.60	141.20	0.76
Respiratory Disease	1046.20	1541.10	1.47
Diabetes Mellitus	58.30	133.70	2.29
Arthritis	138.70	114.40	0.82
Malnutrition	42.00	24.80	0.59
Hypertension	128.80	207.60	1.61
Bronchitis	44.80	62.70	1.40
Heart Disease	29.40	45.70	1.56
Blindness/Deafness	43.00	38.20	0.89
Epilepsy/Mental Retardation	34.50	35.80	1.04
Trauma	45.50	59.10	1.30
Contact with Sharp Object	31.70	34.90	1.10
Twisting or Fracture	36.80	45.30	1.23
Other Injuries	15.70	17.90	1.14

Notes:
a) Places with ≤ 2500 inhabitants
b) Places with > 2500 inhabitants
Source: National Health Survey 1987

Table 3.4 *Relative risk by principal causes of mortality – Teocelo, Mexico 1991: comparison of rates from a rural municipality, Teocelo (14,000 inhabitants) compared with the corresponding national rates*

Causes	Rate[a]	Relative risk[b]
Total	**636.0**	**1.2**
Heart Diseases	137.9	3.9
Respiratory Diseases	91.9	10.3
Diarrhoea and Gastroenteritis	69.0	2.9
Cerebrovascular Diseases	53.6	3.1
Malignant Neoplasms	38.3	1.4
Liver Diseases	38.1	1.6
Nephropathy, Nephrotic and Nephritic Syndrome	30.7	3.0
Accidents	23.0	0.9
Disorders Due to Use of Alcohol	23.0	7.3

Notes:
a) Rates by 100,000 inhabitants
b) Rate for Teocelo/rate for Mexico, see Table 3.2
Source: Municipality of Teocelo, Civil Registration of Deaths

Table 3.5 *Malnutrition rates by region and health service – Chile*

Health service region	Admin region	Population examined	Prevalence of malnutrition Total %	Urban %	Rural %
North	I	31,668	4.1	4.0	6.8
	II	35,170	8.4	8.8	9.8
	III	21,862	9.9	9.0	16.6
	IV	54,433	9.5	8.2	11.2
Centre	V	128,498	8.0	7.4	8.9
Santiago Metropolitan Area	MR	433,501	9.0	8.8	11.0
South	VI	65,514	9.9	9.6	9.9
	VII	91,886	9.5	7.9	10.8
	VIII	173,285	9.2	8.0	11.4
Far South	IX	88,034	8.1	7.9	8.4
	X	96,539	9.0	9.8	9.7
	XI	8,651	7.2	7.0	7.3
	XII	9,065	4.0	4.5	2.9
Total		**1,238,016**	**8.8**	**8.4**	**10.2**

A data set from Mexico illustrates these differences and their relationship to the epidemiological transition. Table 3.2 compares the mortality rates in urban and rural settings. Table 3.3 looks at the morbidity pattern. Taken together, the tables reveal that the relative risk for diarrhoea, pneumonia and malnutrition is higher in rural areas while diabetes mellitus, chronic respiratory diseases, heart diseases and malignant neoplasms are more frequent in urban areas. It is important to note that respiratory diseases are 50 per cent more frequent in urban areas. However, malnutrition is generally higher in rural areas when compared with aggregated urban rates; this is shown in Tables 3.2 and 3.3, and also in Table 3.5, which illustrates a comparable situation in Chile. Table 3.4 compares mortality rates in a town, Teocelo, with the national rates, which are very similar to the rates of Mexico City. People in this town face both high infectious disease rates and high chronic disease rates, as well as an increase in social disease problems, as indicated by the alcohol-related mortality rates – though the accident risk is lower. The data from Teocelo are very typical of a situation of epidemiological transition.

Intra-urban differentials are very much a consequence of population growth and migration. Not only do cities grow globally, but their population profiles change. The understanding of these demographic changes is of crucial importance in order to define strategies for reducing morbidity and mortality and – even more important – for reducing fertility rates. So far hardly any systems or action research has been undertaken in this priority area.

The economic interdependencies between the rural and urban populations are another major feature of the social context of the urban poor, and thus of their health status. Many urban residents in Africa and in many Asian and some Latin American countries have strong ties with rural areas. Investments in urban development can therefore have positive benefits for rural areas. Some residents of peri-urban squatter communities also have houses in rural areas, and many urban communities provide financial support to rural relatives while rural communities supply food to urban areas (see the chapter by Seager). Despite the importance of these interdependencies, there is a striking lack of data and detailed studies on this topic.

Urbanization also leads to complex changes in dependency patterns and ratios in the urban setting. Traditional extended families, characteristic of many rural areas, often break down after a move to an urban area (Figure 3.1). Nuclear households, households as social and economic alliances with members of similar ages and households headed by women are predominant. However, as the duration of residence in urban areas increases, both extended families and nuclear households decrease while female-headed households increase. Alliances, however, remain at similar levels.

Recent arrivals in cities often have high unemployment rates and a few individuals may have to support many people of similar age. Different age-dependency relationships are evident, and breadwinners may suffer from considerable stress. Changes in dependency patterns may expose some groups, such as the elderly and children, to additional risks owing to inadequate family or caretaker support. An understanding of the social patterns outlined above can not only help us to understand the determinants of health status, but is crucial for the design of urban health programmes and targeted health interventions that require the involvement and participation of households.

The features emphasized above are particularly expressed among the poorer strata of any urban population. Rossi-Espagnet et al (1991) and Stephens and Harpham (1991) have pointed out some characteristics that are typical of poor urban areas, and that are different from the rural situation:

- dependence on a cash economy;
- people being forced to settle on land that is environmentally hazardous;
- overcrowding within wards and households;
- insecurity of tenure and, thus, the threat of eviction;
- the breakdown of the traditional family structure; and
- the need for children to work away from the family.

A further set of features of the urban setting relates to the health care delivery and promotion system. These elements and their management are discussed in the chapter by Lorenz and Garner. However, it is important to bear in mind for our discussion of determinants that services are generally easier to provide in urban settings, since the greater population density allows services to be delivered to more people at less cost. Accessibility is often not a crucial determinant. The greater variety of service providers in many urban areas (governmental, NGO, private, traditional) also provides more choices for consumers, which can possibly lead to higher user satisfaction and an increased quality of care and services.

DETERMINANTS OF HEALTH STATUS AND AREAS OF SOCIAL ACTION IN URBAN AREAS

Table 3.6 is an attempt to analyze the urban health problems, their major determinants and the risk groups involved, as well as the potential areas of social action. The Table was constructed by listing urban health problems and examining them with regard to:

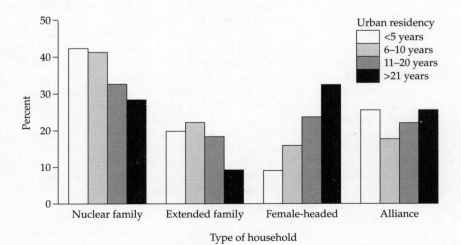

Source: Khayelitsha, Cape Town (Pick, W, 1992)

Figure 3.1 *Household composition during urbanization – Khayelitsha, Cape Town*

- Occurrence by level of urbanization, based on the classification by the World Bank (1991)

Group 1:   Heavily urbanized countries with more than 75 per cent of the people living in cities (usually including megacities), but where rates of urban growth are declining. Most growth is attributable to natural increase rather than migration. Typical of Latin America eg Argentina, Mexico, Colombia, Brazil.

Group 2:   Recently urbanized, with about half the population living in urban areas. Growth rates have peaked and are beginning to decline. Typical of North African and some Asian countries eg Algeria, Morocco, Malaysia.

Group 3:   Primarily rural but rapidly urbanizing. Migration a major source of urban growth, although predominantly male migration has been replaced by household migration, leading to a shift towards natural increase as the major cause of growth. Typical of African countries eg Senegal, Ivory Coast, Nigeria, Sudan, Kenya, Zaire.

Group 4:   Large, mostly rural countries. Major urban concentrations. Urban growth rates stabilized at high levels and projected to continue for next decade. Typical of large Asian countries eg India, Indonesia, China.

- Determinants of disease in terms of environmental, biological, social and economic factors
- Risk groups: specifically the urban poor and sub-groups within the urban poor
- Priority for intervention as defined in Table 3.6
- Actions required, according to the sector which would have the main responsibility for the action
- Specific target groups for interventions, where these differ from those affected by the disease

The summary presented in Table 3.6 deliberately avoids offering suggestions for the priority to be assigned to each disease or condition. Various methods have been proposed for setting priorities for public health interventions (as reviewed in Feachem et al 1989, Jamison et al 1993 and World Bank 1993). Morbidity and mortality burdens are obvious criteria, but tried and proven interventions are equally important. In many cases the interventions with the maximum potential cost-benefit will be the ones that must be selected. Newer standardized approaches based on disability adjusted life years (DALYs, Murray 1994, Murray and Lopez 1994) have been established in conjunction with the World Development Report 1993 (World Bank 1993, Murray et al 1994) and offer the basis for comparative priority setting across different conditions. However, they are still very much based on the professional, technical assessment of the value of morbidity and disability, ie they are based on normative needs. The perceptions of those concerned and affected is not taken into account, although these perceptions can represent a major determinant for reaching a consensus on priorities and subsequent actions (Tanner 1989, and the chapter by Lorenz and Garner). The extension of the DALY concept from its current disease or condition basis to a risk based approach (Murray et al 1994) will therefore offer attractive opportunities, particularly for the comprehensive planning of urban health development programmes.

Table 3.6 *Urban health status: priority conditions, determinants and possible actions by sectors*

Conditions	Level[a]	Determinants[b]	
Diarrhoeal diseases	1–4	Water, sanitation, hygiene behaviour	
Respiratory diseases Acute respiratory infections			
Pneumonia	1–4	Indoor air pollution, outdoor air pollution, crowding	
Tuberculosis	2–4	Indoor air pollution, outdoor air pollution, crowding	
Chronic respiratory disease	1–4	Overcrowding, poor immune status, air pollution, housing	
Sexually-transmitted disease	1–4	Changing social context	
AIDS		Changing social context	
Measles	1–4	Overcrowding, poor immune status	
Helminths	1–4	Water, sanitation, hygiene behaviour	
Malaria	2–4	Housing, drainage, climate	
Obstetric deaths	1–4	ANC, abortion legislation, education	
Perinatal deaths	1–4	ANC, education	
Cancer	1–4	Lifestyle: smoking, diet	
Cervical cancer		Parity, STD	
Cardiovascular diseases	1–4	Lifestyle: smoking, diet, exercise	
Trauma			
Traffic	1–4	Transport facilities/infrastructure	
Occupational	1–4	Legislation, education	
Violence	1–4	Alcohol, drugs, social factors	
Household accidents	1–4	Housing and living conditions	
Mental and behavioural diseases/Addictions	1–4	Changing social context, stress/life events, lacking social supports	
Alcoholism	1–4	Stress/life events, lacking social supports	
Drug addiction	1–4	Availability, stress/life events, lacking social supports	
Malnutrition	1–4	Poverty, education, food availability and access	
Skin disease	1–4	Water sanitation, hygiene behaviour and housing	
Diarrhoeal diseases	Children <5	Provision of water, sanitation, education control[c]	Children <5 Mothers/ carers

Table 3.6 *Continued*

Conditions	Risk groups[a]	Action by sector[b]	Target group
Respiratory diseases			
Acute respiratory infections	Children	Housing, legislation, education, infra-structure, control	Children, Carers
Pneumonia			
Tuberculosis	Adults	Control	Adults
Chronic respiratory disease	All	Legislation, control	All
Sexually-transmitted disease	Adults	Education, control	Youth, adults
AIDS	Adults	Education, control	Youth, adults
Measles	Children <5	Control	Children <5
Helminths	Children <5	Control, provision of sanitation, water, education	Children/ adults
Malaria	Children <5 Adults (migrants)	Housing, infra-structure, control	All
Obstetric deaths	Women-RA	Legislation, control	Women-RA
Perinatal deaths	Women-RA	Control	Women-RA
Cancer	Adult	Control, education	All
Cervical cancer	Women-RA	Control, education	Women-RA
Cardiovascular diseases	Adults	Control, education	All
Trauma			
Traffic	All	Legislation, education,	All
Occupational	Workers	infrastructure	Workers
Violence	All	Legislation, education,	employers
Household accidents	Children	Social support, legislation	All
		Housing, education	All
Mental and behav-ioural diseases	All	Social support	All
Addictions	Adults	Social support	>5 years
Alcoholism	Youth and adults	Social support	>5 years
Drug addiction			
Malnutrition	Children <5	Education, control, supply[d]	Mothers, Children
Skin disease	Children and youth	Control	Children, Mothers

Notes:
a) Level of urbanization; classification based on World Bank (1991)
b) Poverty and lack of primary education are determinants for all conditions and, thus, not specifically included in all boxes. When education is specified as determinant, it points at the lack of specific information and education in the respective field.
c) Control entails preventive and curative actions by the health services
d) Supply entails direct food supply and/or finances
Women-RA/Women of Reproductive Age
ANC   Antenatal care

Table 3.7 *Determinants of health status: the role of migration compared with social and economic status*

Factors associated with maternal mental disorders in Rio de Janeiro

Variable	Number of subject	Subject with mental disorder %	Relative risk
Income per capita			
Lowest 25%	112	47.3	1.6
Middle 50%	225	33.8	1.1*
Highest 25%	123	30.3	1.0
Environmental conditions			
Bad (score 0–8)	87	48.3	1.4
Moderate (score 9–13)	233	33.1	0.95*
Good (score 14–17)	138	15.0	1.0
Mother's education			
Unschooled	263	40.7	1.3
Schooled	195	30.7	1.0*
Mother's age			
Teenager (<20 years)	31	35.5	0.97
Non-teenager (20+ years)	428	36.4	1.0
Marital status			
Partnerless	72	45.8	1.4
Living with partner	376	34.0	1.0
Parity			
≥3 children	172	41.3	1.4
2–3 children	136	36.0	1.2
1 child	145	30.3	1.1
Mother's length of residence in Rocinha			
≤3 years (recent migrant)	109	37.6	1.2
4–9 years (intermediate migrant)	137	40.1	1.3
≥10 years (long term migrant)	117	35.0	1.1
Locally born	96	31.2	1.0

Notes:
* Statistically significant associations – P < 0.05
Source: Data from Reichenheim and Harpham (1991)

Three groups of determinants immediately emerge: socio-behavioural factors, environmental factors and the factors related to the delivery of social services. Poverty and lack of primary education are major determinants of ill health in rural and urban settings. As they apply to all diseases and conditions, they are not specifically listed in Table 3.6. The spectrum of diseases and conditions further reveals the importance of the epidemiological transition in the urban context in developing countries. Particular attention needs to be paid to the environmental determinants and conditions that affect the health status of the populations. Hardoy et al (1990), Hardoy and Satterthwaite (1992), Bradley et al (1992) and the *World Development Report 1992* (World Bank 1992) have comprehensively reviewed various aspects of the interactions between environment, health and social development within the urban context.

Urbanization is characterized by a high degree of mobility of the population, mainly reflected in high migration rates. The role of migration as a determinant of ill health needs special attention. Recent data, however, indicate that migration may be a less important determinant than socioeconomic status, as illustrated by a study in the largest squatter area of Rio de Janeiro, Rocinha (Reichenheim and Harpham 1991). Table 3.7 summarizes the main findings of this study, which examined the role of migration with regard to maternal mental health. In conclusion, these observations and the summary presented in Table 3.6 emphasize that economic development and social support activities need to be an integral part of urban health development planning and the resulting programmes.

CONCLUSION

The review of the features and the determinants of urban health status leads to a series of conclusions and recommendations that could be of importance for the planning and implementation of urban health development programmes.

1. Urban health problems are too large, and the underlying determinants are too complex, for them to be managed by Ministries of Health alone. This implies that different sectors will need to take joint or full responsibility, depending on the specific problem. For example, the agricultural sector for dietary components; the housing sector for shelter, housing and sanitation; the education and communication sectors for health education and information components; the energy sector for pollution control; the transport sector for traffic safety; the industrial sector for pollution control and control of occupational hazards; and the community development sector for health promotion and community involvement components.

It is evident that this truly multisectoral approach implies that governments must ensure the establishment of coordinating bodies for urban health activities. Experience at this level is further illustrated in the chapters by Goldstein et al and Hecht. Legislation and government supervision should ensure a minimum standard of service provision by all service providers in the social sector.

The overall approach in an urban health development programme needs to respect the primary health care strategy, which also calls for a highly multisectoral, non-medicalized approach. In all these efforts, decentralization of primary health care services should be the guiding strategy, which implies that resources and autonomy must be given to local authorities. This in turn may improve accessibility and community participation in particular, and efficiency of the programmes in general.

2. Social support programmes should be considered as a main strategy for addressing social conditions leading to ill health, such as mental problems, addictions, violence and teenage pregnancy. These programmes, combined with investments in infrastructure through the housing sector, will remain the backbone of attempts to improve the health status of urban populations.

3. Medium sized cities (up to five million inhabitants) should also become a priority target for urban health interventions. This recommendation emerges mainly from the Latin American experience. Medium sized cities show growth rates and health indicators comparable to those of megacities (> five million inhabitants), but it may be easier to design cost-effective interventions for them, because of easier access and because they often show less social stratification. Whether this holds true for the Asian and African contexts needs to be established and merits further attention.

4. Identification of target groups according to risk profiles established with standardized procedures for setting priorities should remain the basis for interventions, but besides biological factors these procedures must include the full range of psychosocial risks, particularly teenage pregnancy, alcohol and drug abuse.

5. Approaches to controlling air and noise pollution should receive high priority in municipal health plans, given the substantial environmental health impacts (Bradley et al 1992). These approaches should complement efforts in communicable disease control.

6. Education and health promotion programmes should incorporate components designed to trigger changes in aspects of lifestyle that are major determinants of urban health problems. This becomes particularly important for the control of chronic illnesses and adult health problems. Therefore Information Education Communication (IEC) and health promotion must be an integral part of action to improve the health status of urban populations.

7. Data collection and its effective use as part of the health management system are particularly deficient in urban settings. Research projects, and evaluations of urban health programmes, need to focus on obtaining disaggregated data to reveal intra-urban differentials across social and economic groups which will allow the identification of high risk groups and provide the basis for more rational priority setting processes, which in turn may lead to more equitable approaches in health care delivery and health promotion.

This set of conclusions and recommendations clearly indicates that the tools for action are already known and available. However, it further shows us that it will not be simple for an urban health development programme to adopt these available technical solutions, which range, for example, from housing to immunization or micronutrient supplementation programmes. Besides substantial policy changes and a sustained commitment to alleviating poverty, concepts and strategies are needed which are precisely tailored to each setting. This applies not only to the content but also to the implementation arrangements. While the careful consideration of the former is generally advocated, and has been realized in most programmes, the latter is often neglected. Implementation arrangements include the careful definition of responsibility and authority at each level of action and among each of the institutions or bodies involved. Besides sound concepts and well-defined strategies oriented to particular risk groups, it is this process that will create and define commitment and will therefore become the most crucial determinant in our attempts to tackle and reduce the problems that result in the urban poor suffering from having 'the worst of both worlds' – both the underdeveloped and the modern ones.

REFERENCES

Bradley, D Cairncross, S Harpham, T and Stephens, C (1992) *A Review of Environmental Health Impacts in Developing Country Cities* Urban Management Program Paper 6, World Bank, Washington DC

Feachem, R Graham, W and Timaeus, I (1989) Identifying Health Problems and Health Research Priorities in Developing Countries *Journal of Tropical Medicine and Hygiene*, 91, pp 133–191

Hardoy, J and Satterthwaite, D (1992) *Environmental Problems in Third World Cities: an Agenda for the Poor and the Planet* International Institute for Environment and Development, London

Hardoy, J Cairncross, S and Satterthwaite, D (1990) *The Poor Die Young: Housing and Health in Third World Cities* Earthscan, London

Harpham, T Lusty, T and Vaughan, P (1988) *In the Shadow of the City: Community Health and the Urban Poor* Oxford University Press, Oxford

Jamison, D Mosley, W Measham, A and Bobadilla, J (1993) *Disease Control Priorities in Developing Countries* Oxford University Press, Oxford

Murray, C (1994) Quantifying the Burden of Disease: the Technical Basis for Disability Adjusted Life Years *Bulletin of the World Health Organization*, 72, pp 429–445

Murray, C and Lopez, A (1994) Quantifying Disability: Data, Methods and Results *Bulletin of the World Health Organization*, 72, pp 481–494

Murray, C Lopez, A and Jamison, D (1994) The Global Burden of Disease in 1990: Summary Results, Sensitivity Analysis and Future Directions *Bulletin of the World Health Organization*, 72, pp 495–509

Pick, W (1991) *Urbanization and Women's Health in Cape Town, South Africa* Research Paper 58, Takemi Programme in International Health, Harvard School of Public Health (unpublished)

Reichenheim, M and Harpham, T (1991) Maternal Mental Health in a Squatter Settlement of Rio de Janeiro *British Journal of Psychiatry*, 155, pp 44–47

Rossi-Espagnet, A Goldstein, G and Tabibzadeh, I (1991) Urbanization and Health in Developing Countries: Challenge for Health for All *World Health Statistics Quarterly*, 44, pp 187–244

Stephens, C and Harpham, T (1991) *Slum Improvement: Health Improvement?* Health Policy Unit, London School of Hygiene and Tropical Medicine, London

Stephens, C Timaeus, I Ackerman, M et al (1994) *Environment amd Health in Developing Countries: an Analysis of Intra-urban Differentials using Existing Data* London School of Hygiene and Tropical Medicine, London

Tanner, M (1989) From the Bench to the Field – Control of Parasitic Infections within Primary Health Care *Parasitology*, 99, pp S81–S92

World Bank (1991) *Urban Policy and Economic Development: Agenda for the 1990s* World Bank, Washington DC

World Bank (1992) *World Development Report 1992 – Development and the Environment* Oxford University Press, Oxford

World Bank (1993) *World Development Report 1993 – Investing in Health* Oxford University Press, Oxford

World Health Organization (1992) *Report on Urbanization* WHO Commission on Health and Environment

4

Organizing and Managing Urban Health Services

Nick Lorenz and Paul Garner (eds)

INTRODUCTION

In urban areas there is usually a mix of providers offering various health services. There may be government services run by the local council, municipal council, state or central ministry; private (for profit) hospitals, laboratories and practitioners; and a variety of nongovernment providers, including missions and charities. Given these complex circumstances, senior health managers have to decide exactly what the responsibilities of the state are in public health, and in ensuring access of urban populations to health services. They need to examine what minimum standards of care are appropriate for the population; what changes in the organizational design of government are needed to increase the effectiveness of government health services; and the appropriate changes in the relationship between the government and the private sector. The complexity of the existing pattern of provision and financing means that planning cannot be prescriptive. Rather, managers must take account of the particular political environment they are working in, and the established relationships within organizations and between different providers. Thus managers have to examine ways of improving their effectiveness within their current environment, as well as acting as agents of change to the existing system where the opportunities arise.

While acknowledging the importance of broader public health issues, such as problems related to water, sanitation or mass campaigns to promote healthy lifestyles, it is not possible to cover these issues here. Financing is not dealt with here, but is covered in the chapter by Thomas and McPake. In this chapter we focus on clinical health services, that is, curative and preventive health services, that consist of contact between a health worker and a patient. This includes public health programmes implemented through health service providers.

* Based on contributions by Antoine Degrémont, Lilia Duran Gonzalez, Emile Jeannée, Ashok Yesudian
** Thanks to Sara Bennett of the London School of Hygiene and Tropical Medicine for helpful and constructive comments on an earlier version of this chapter

EFFECTIVE PLANNING

Situation

Health service planners often form strategies without analysis of the current provider environment. They risk making the wrong assumptions about the type of services that must be provided, or plans for services that are incompatible with existing provision financing. A more fundamental overview of what the government is trying to do with respect to health service provision is needed to formulate appropriate long term plans. This will require formulation of explicit goals and objectives, stated in managerial (rather than epidemiological) terms, compatible with existing government policies.

Often a blueprint approach to planning is taken: that services should conform to certain standard staffing, activity or equipment guidelines. This simple method may help, but is often thwarted for several reasons. Firstly, the standards set may be out of date or too high for the recurrent resource base of the country. Secondly, the blueprint does not take into account the authority or lack of it between the government manager and the health provider. What, for example, can a national health department do about the standards of care provided in a municipal hospital? Thirdly, blueprint approaches smack of a centralized approach, not taking into account local epidemiological and social factors influencing disease patterns and service utilization. Nor does this facilitate local innovation and adaptation, such as trying out different approaches to provide health care for adolescents. Finally, blueprint approaches may be so inflexible and developed by those with limited influence over the system, that when services do not reach the standards set, nobody does anything about it.

Yet the very milieu that makes the blueprint approach inappropriate also means that senior health managers need a very clear vision of what they are aiming to achieve. This requires an understanding of the existing pattern of provision, and a clarity of purpose for the future. Without this, planning and management will be piecemeal and *ad hoc*.

Possible solutions

At a city level, there is a need for a comprehensive assessment of current provision, and formulation of a health service strategy. This may be done by the Ministry of Health, or in cities where provision has been devolved to the city, by the Municipality. There are many different techniques for planning, and the steps given below are adapted from Gordon et al 1990. The process is illustrative of one approach managers can take in formulating clearly the policy, goals, objectives and strategy in planning, and assumes service provision is the responsibility of the Municipality.

The starting point for the planning process is to **identify the guiding principles** of the Municipality. If these are not explicit, they need to be formulated and drafted. For example, is a guiding principle equity of access, ensuring a simple, basic minimum package of health care is accessible to all? Is collaboration between health and other sectors, such as education, a guiding principle?

A crucial element is the **purpose** of the Municipality. Is it to provide appropriate and affordable primary health services for the entire city population? Or is it to provide for the poor, and to facilitate private service provision for higher income groups?

Planners need to assess the **internal environment** with respect to resources available (for example staff, money and infrastructure). The current structure and stated function of government services, particularly with respect to the various service tiers, needs careful delineating (see 'government health services' below).

The planners should evaluate the **external environment**. This includes the current national policy with respect to direct provision of service compared with promoting or regulating the private sector; the direction of decentralization; national policy for health sector financing; national norms setting service standards or configurations; and the level of flexibility the Municipality has in interpreting these policies (see 'decentralization' and 'private providers' below).

This information should provide a sufficient basis to form a realistic strategic plan, consisting of the **goals of the organization, and broad objectives** by which these goals will be strived for.

One of the problems with health service planning in the past is that goals and objectives are stated in highly specific, epidemiological terms. Determinants of health status, as measured through epidemiological parameters, are frequently outside of the health service sector (McKeown 1979). Whilst it is appropriate to strive for improvements in health status, more realistic objectives (that are achievable, measurable and time specific) are more useful in improving management.

Finally, this process leads to a series of detailed plans based on **operational objectives** that are formulated in the process of deciding what is needed to pursue the strategic objectives. These require detailed information about existing health services and indicators of need and demand.

There are four key areas that planners should consider carefully as they formulate their goals and strategy. These are: current decentralization policies altering government administrative structures; the debate over government health service tiers; the relationship between the government and the private sector; and institutional development to improve managerial capacity in government health services. There are many excellent texts covering broader planning concerns (for example, Lee and Mills 1982, Segall 1991).

DECENTRALIZATION OF GOVERNMENT SERVICES

Situation

Decentralization of power, resources and administration from national bodies to municipal and submunicipal levels has been advocated as cities grow in size and as the public functions of government become increasingly complex. It makes sense that increases in size and complexity require decentralization to maintain managerial efficiency, and this fits with contingency theory with respect to organizational design (Child 1984). Indeed, it is common sense that public services such as solid waste disposal are organized within a city or by locality, and not by ministries external to the city. Local control of services is also seen as an important way of ensuring coordination between different government sectors to promote intersectoral action with its consequent beneficial effect on people's health.

Political forces in favour of decentralization are particularly powerful in urban areas: the populations served by local authorities are large, politically sensitized and often geographically adjacent to national decision makers. Theoretically, devolution of power should increase the accountability of public services to those they serve. The disadvantage is that services are more vulnerable to short term political influences. However, the level, extent and nature of decentralization varies between countries and cities (Mills et al 1990 and Gilson et al in press). Table 4.1 is a qualitative, subjective assessment by urban managers from different cities.

If there are so many advantages of decentralization, why is the degree to which it has occurred so variable? Partly this is because decentralization is a much more complex process than it first appears, and means different things in different cities and for different policy strategists. Devolution, the most extreme form of decentralization, implies local financial autonomy. Few central ministries will hand over resources without controlling how they are spent. 'Poor' cities, highly dependent on central funds, find it difficult to become autonomous, and are likely to remain partly controlled by national ministries who authorize their budgets. This causes a curious management phenomenon of upside down delegation where the wrong things are delegated. The very least the centre should do is delegate authority, whilst remaining ultimately responsible and accountable. Instead, responsibility is delegated but the authority and decision making remains central. It is hardly surprising in these circumstances that accountability is ambiguous (Kanji, personal communication).

Table 4.1 *Examples of decentralization in different cities*

Area of decentralization	Bombay	Dar es Salaam	Mexico City	Cape Town
Political will for decentralization	+	++	++	+++
Legal framework for decentralization	+	++	+++	+++
Degree of implementation of decentralization	+	+	−	++
Planning capacities of local government	++	+	+++	++
Management capacities of local government	++	+	+++	+++
Actual power of local government to take decisions	+	−	+	++
Accountability to higher levels	+++	+++	+++	+
Accountability to the population	+	+	++	−
Locally generated funds administered locally	++	+	+	−
Central fund allocation	++	+++	+++	+++

Source: Participants at 'Consultation on urban health', Eggiwil, Switzerland 1992
+++ high   ++ medium   + little   − very little or non existent

Some cities are so big that decentralization to a municipal level may still mean a centralized bureaucratic approach, as there is decentralization of decision making to a local level, or a capacity for intersectoral collaboration at the point of delivery. For example, district decentralization in Mexico means administrative units for two million people per district.

Possibilities of intersectoral collaboration are further compromised by the fact that sectoral vertical organization continues, despite the rhetoric, as that is how the organizations are used to functioning. In fact, divisions between sectors may be so marked that the process of decentralization occurs independently within sectors, with no reference or linkage to other government ministries.

Possible solutions

Decentralization to municipal or lower levels is theoretically a positive move to improve health status and service delivery in a city. However, to do this municipalities need: resources (discussed in the chapter by Thomas and McPake); power to make decisions; and a capacity to plan and manage. This requires: political will; an organizational structure that is sufficiently flexible and relatively free of bureaucratic constraints to allow decision making by managers; information on which to base rational decisions; power over professional groups, particularly doctors; and managerial skills (discussed below).

In countries with a high level of local autonomy, intersectoral plans and working relationships at a municipal level need drawing up early in the life of the municipality. In countries where there is still some central influence over municipal planning, intersectoral approaches at municipal level will be difficult in the absence of intersectoral policies at higher or national levels. In slum areas, it is particularly important to ensure coordination between sectors occurs close to the point of service delivery. This may mean local offices or mechanisms of communication between sectors and in dialogue with politicians and local communities.

GOVERNMENT HEALTH SERVICE TIERS

Situation

There is considerable debate concerning the role of hospitals in urban health services (Ebrahim and Ranken 1988, Anon 1993). In cities there is usually already a mix of facilities: the planner needs to evaluate the *balance of various tiers*, how much each receives, what they do and their responsibilities in providing or supervising outreach services in their catchment area. The planner can then modify resource allocation in pursuit of an equitable, efficient, effective health service (Mills 1990a, Mills 1990b).

In many countries the health system attempts to ration scarce and expensive services by distancing them from direct contact with the patient through intermediate service tiers. The theory is that most patients can be provided for at basic facilities, and that those requiring more sophisticated care can be referred on to higher levels in the system.

In practice, however, lower service tiers are often underused due to shortages of drugs and a reputation for poor quality care. The referral process is a technique of rational resource use in the mind of the planner but of little relevance to the user. People make rational decisions about where they want to go: this means that they may use higher tiers in the system as first points of contact. This is often termed 'misuse', which suggests malicious intent on the part of the patient. This is inaccurate: managers need to examine why the system does not perform as they expect it to.

The epidemiological and demographic transition is also causing confusion with respect to care given at basic health facilities. In the past, diseases of the transition were relatively uncommon and seen as the traditional province of doctors, whilst responsibility for the common diseases, including life threatening conditions such as pneumonia, was delegated to paramedics. In addition, the long term treatment required for many 'transition' diseases has substantial resource implications: can governments afford to pay for the long term care needed? Will this mean insufficient resources to treat acute infectious diseases?

There are *differences in the meaning* of standard terminology when comparing health service mixes between countries. This affects comprehension when people with different experiences are comparing service tiers. For example, a health centre in one country may be performing the same functions as a district hospital in another country. To assist in cross-country comparisons, we have classed services into four tiers (Table 4.2).

There remain the comparisons between countries: if urban health services in different cities are matched against the tier model, it can be seen that a gap at tier two occurs in a number of countries (Table 4.3). This seems odd. History may reveal the explanation: specialist city hospitals were built prior to the widespread adoption of the district health service approach, where the hospital is responsible for community health

Table 4.2 *Terminology for health service tiers*

Tier/ level	Common terminology	Content	Country examples
1	Primary	First contact/ minimum package	Dispensary (Tanzania) Aid post (Papua New Guinea)
2	Advanced primary	Manage referrals supervision of tier 1, inpatients, trauma, outpatients, in-patient obstetric care	Health centre (Tanzania) Reference centre (Mexico) District hospital (Thailand)
3	Secondary	Major inpatient care, resident specialists	District hospital (Pakistan)
4	Tertiary	Highly specialized care, national medical teaching institutions	Specialist hospital, regional hospital, teaching hospital

Table 4.3 *Tiers in the government health system: some cities compared*

Tier of care	Content (see Table 4.2)	City examples Teocelo, Mexico	Bombay, India	Ouagadougou, Burkina Faso
1	Minimum package	Community health module	Health post, Dispensary, Maternity homes	Centre for health and social promotion, maternity
2	First referral, supervision, some inpatients	Advanced unit for comprehensive health care	None	None
3	Major inpatient care, basic specialist care	Secondary hospital	General hospital	None
4	Highest level of medical care available in the city	Centre of medical specialities	Teaching hospital	National hospital

services in a defined catchment area and provides less specialist medical care than the big urban centres (King 1966). Primary health care stressed low cost accessible basic services with little reference to hospitals. The result is cities with tier one, but an absent tier two. In addition, strategic planning has often been absent as urban populations have expanded. Low cost tier one facilities may have been built, but without appropriate clinical support or inpatient facilities.

Possible solutions

New service tiers
The gap in service tiers in urban areas has led some countries to build tier two facilities in urban areas (World Health Organization 1991). The WHO is now promoting this approach (World Health Organization 1992). Much of the impetus for this idea comes from successes in Cali (Shepard et al 1993) and Mexico (González et al 1992). However, questions have been raised concerning its widespread adoption (Anon 1993). In one sub-Saharan African country, a World Bank loan was being used to build 'reference centres' in a health system where the main problems were caused by a weak managerial environment, not a lack of capital investment (Box 4.1); indeed, the country did not have the medical staff or recurrent budget to cover the costs of the new facilities.

'Reference centres' assume patients behave in a way that health planners expect of them: that is, they first go to the primary level facility, and are then referred upwards. Anyone working in health services

---

Box 4.1

DO URBAN HEALTH SERVICES NEED NEW FACILITIES OR BETTER MANAGEMENT?

In Maseru, the national hospital was reported to be overused and the urban health centres of poor quality and low throughput. The Ministry of Health decided to build 'reference centres' using a loan from the World Bank to solve these problems. However, research showed:

- utilization levels per clinician at the hospital were similar to the health centres;
- the perception of overuse at the hospital was caused by poor patient flow;
- the clinical care provided at the hospital was no better than that at health centres;
- hospital outpatient department average costs were 40 per cent greater than at health centres, which was much less than anticipated.

The planning implications of the study showed that there were major national management issues to tackle in improving the health system overall. Building new service tiers was unlikely to change anything, and the recurrent budget shortfall meant the MOH did not have the resources to run the new clinics. In fact, three centres had already been built over the last five years in the city and never opened.

Source: Pepperall and Garner (1992), Holdsworth et al (1994)

---

realizes this is rarely the case, and people decide where they wish to go. If reference centres do provide better care, it is likely that patients will choose to use them in preference to the health centres. There needs to be some mechanism to ensure staff at the reference centres are made responsible for the work of the health centres, so that they ensure the staff are providing good quality care at adjacent clinics, and not just in their own facility.

Although WHO claims these centres are not district hospitals (Ashton 1993), the debate reflects the confusion over terminology rather than function outlined earlier. Reference centres clearly fulfil the role of tier two facilities, take inpatients and are responsible for community health in a defined geographic area. As such, staffing patterns (including the need for night cover and staff housing) have to be considered in building estimates and projected recurrent costs of running them. What is important about WHO's re-affirmation of the district health service approach is that it reminds planners that hospitals should have a geographically defined catchment population to whom they have responsibility with respect to managing primary health services.

Reallocation of resources

Tier three facilities (larger hospitals) remain extremely costly to run, and yet little is known about their output and coverage ie their effectiveness (Mills 1990a). If countries decide to improve their primary health service within a fixed budget, then the additional resources will need to come from somewhere. It is possible that more efficient use of the resources available would be achieved by constraining or even reducing the cost of hospitals, and reallocating the money and people to primary health services. Alternatively, if governments have an expanding recurrent budget for health care provision, planners could ensure lower tier services have a greater proportion of the increment (Segall 1991). This will require strong political will, active management and decentralized systems of resource allocation. If public expenditure on services at tiers three and four is constrained by freezing current allocations, these levels could develop their own sources of incomes which is then used and managed within the facility for assisting with recurrent costs. In the interim, managers could devise systems to ensure the medical expertise at tier three is used to provide clinical support to staff in tier two facilities.

Care of diseases of the transition

The assumption that diseases of the transition need a higher level of medical care than infectious diseases in rural areas needs questioning. At its simplest, the assumption implies that an adult with hypertension needs a higher level of medical expertise than a child with severe pneumonia. In fact, the bulk of diseases of the transition can be provided at tier one and do not require sophisticated technology. However, professionals at tiers two and three will need to set standard protocols for care, and provide supervision of training of health workers at tier one. This may require diagnosis, treatment initiation and occasional follow up at tiers two and three (Box 4.3).

Box 4.2

REVENUE RAISING IN HOSPITALS

In the UK, one aspect of current national policy aims to increase hospital efficiency by encouraging hospitals to become budget holders. Hospitals thus become more autonomous, and are given a budget with which there is much greater flexibility for local decisions about how resources are used within the hospital. Some hospitals have started their own income generating schemes, both through cross-subsidisation of public services with private service fees, and through commercial ventures within the hospitals, such as small shops.

Foster professional respectability of primary care

Professional and public respectability and credibility of primary care, particularly at tiers one and two in the health system, is low. Preventive and public health generally is regarded as the poor relation to the high technology of hospital care. This process of development will require the following actions:

- Foster education and training of health professionals at undergraduate and postgraduate levels in primary level care and public health.
- Ensure postgraduate training in these fields is linked to a career structure with pay and conditions of service at least equivalent to that of hospital clinicians.

Box 4.3

TREATING HYPERTENSION IN PIKINE

Hypertension is a common medical problem in Pikine, a suburb of Dakar in Senegal with 650,000 inhabitants. Studies in selected groups of salaried persons have shown prevalences of arterial hypertension (according to WHO definition) of up to 7.4 per cent in men and 10.2 per cent in women.

The medicosocial support is provided through baseline health facilities, where paramedical staff are working. At this level not only the case finding takes place but also the follow up of confirmed cases of hypertension. The paramedical staff of this level of care supervise the compliance of the patients and detect treatment failures and problems related to the disease.

The referral level with a general practitioner confirms the diagnosis, chooses the appropriate treatment and takes care of referred cases of arterial hypertension. This level also ensures quality of care of the baseline health facilities through continuous supervision.

Source: Astagneau et al (1992)

- In-service training for staff already working in levels one and two in primary health care and public health.
- Promotion of the value of levels one and two through publicity of flagship units such as those in Mexico (Box 4.4).
- Ensure active involvement of senior clinicians in the approach taken by levels one and two by including primary health care teaching and supervision responsibilities in their job description.

Box 4.4

COMPREHENSIVE HEALTH CARE IN MEXICO

In the Teocelo Advanced Unit for comprehensive health care (300 km from Mexico City) the School of Public Health organizes a residential Masters programme in Population Mental Health for psychologists, social workers and physicians. There is a joint support from both the School of Public Health and the Ministry of Health. Also, part of the training for specialists in surgery and anaesthesiology takes place in this unit under the supervision of the University of Veracruz. Undergraduate students (psychology, medicine, dentistry, nursing) are trained in a multiprofessional approach to advance teamwork. The National Autonomous University of Mexico supports this programme. Inservice training for physicians working at the unit is offered following the residential programme for family medicine. The nurses working within the network of the governmental health system also receive regular inservice training, with an emphasis on public health issues. The medical staff has the opportunity for telephonic consultation with the National Institute of Paediatrics.

RELATIONSHIP WITH PRIVATE PROVIDERS

Situation

In some cities, the private (for profit and not for profit) sector is a main provider of curative first contact care. This is typical in many Asian cities, where the main providers of care in poor areas are private practitioners (Garner and Thaver 1993). International agencies and governments are examining ways in which care provision through the private sector can be enabled (World Bank 1993). However, this is more complicated than it first appears.

Doctors are responsible for creating demands for health care (Klein 1993), and private providers are motivated by profit. Thus the objective of the state in ensuring health services are available to the population is different from that of the private provider, whose main objective is profit. This 'principal agent problem' requires structures to ensure that the objectives of the agent (the private provider) and the principal (the state) are made more compatible. This requires a complex mix of effective regulation and financial incentives, many of which are currently not in place or only partially working (Bennett et al 1994).

Establishing a relationship between existing autonomous providers and the state is fraught with difficulties, and there are particular problems with government officers working in private practice (see for example, Hülsebusch 1993).

The quality of care of private providers varies a lot from very high to very low. In low income urban areas care is often of low quality. Whilst private providers may be more polite to their patients, the technical quality of their care is not necessarily better. In Dar es Salaam basic outpatient care provided in the voluntary and government sector was compared. The proportion of consultations where a potentially serious error was made was virtually the same between the two types of providers. However, voluntary providers spent longer with their patients, and treated them in a more humane way (Kanji et al in press).

Whilst private providers are seen as a good way of reducing direct state responsibility for health care, there are a number of problems with private providers providing care. Private providers are driven by market forces: thus services which are not profitable are neglected. In particular, preventive interventions, or interventions whose effect is on the community rather than the individual, are likely to be ignored. Secondly, private providers may not operate to maximum allocative efficiency, and overprovide services. Thirdly, a purely market approach to care provision compromises equity of access to basic services. Chronic diseases such as diabetes will *a priori* be less attractive for the private sector as the necessary resources to afford such care will not be accessible for all the population in need. The issues are complex and are discussed elsewhere (Bennett 1992, Bennett et al 1994).

Possible solutions

As already stated earlier in this chapter effective planning requires governments to decide on precisely what their principles and objectives are. Many governments may consider that their responsibility in health services is to ensure the availability of services at tiers one and two to the whole population. Most countries will view tier three as a government responsibility: this needs careful review against the resources available. Often tier three is provided, but is not accessible to a large proportion of the population. It may be that countries prioritize a minimum package accessible to all (World Bank 1993). Yet enabling private care to expand is a relatively easy process for governments. Regulating it is more difficult.

Though health care provision is in some respects a product as any other, there are fundamental differences. To begin with, health care is important as it relieves suffering (Normand 1991). Secondly, health care can be dangerous, especially if inappropriate therapies are given or care is not delivered properly. Governments, then, have a definite responsibility to ensure a minimum quality of care to protect the population from the adverse effects of health care. This requires minimal basic care standards, package of activities and coverage including maximum fees for services. Regulation requires legislation; implementation procedures; information systems; monitoring mechanisms; and effective and rapid procedures. The role of the press and the community in highlighting poor practice should not be underestimated, but is unlikely to be a viable process in autocratic societies.

There is much debate about government regulation through professional bodies. Even when the function and activities of the professional body are set by the government, the organization is often run by doctors, with substantial vested interests in favour of the profession even when this is not in the best interests of the consumer or government (Bennett et al 1994). Medical professionals often have powerful professional associations (equivalent to trade unions) with a number of functions representing the interests of members (Box 4.5).

One area worthy of further exploration in cities where private practice is already well established are systems of voluntary accreditation by the government. Facilities can ask the government to consider them for accreditation: if they pass the various criteria and inspections, they become accredited providers of a particular type or level of care. This requires inspection for renewal. The advantage for the provider is that accreditation may increase their market advantage (Box 4.6).

THE AGENTS OF CHANGE

Situation

Management and planning in urban health services requires skilled personnel at policy level capable of analyzing the current political, financial and policy factors; restructuring health service financing and management to increase efficiency; and making the best use of resources available. Most health managers are doctors, and the management demands on them go far beyond their capacities. Managers are required at lower levels in the system, at municipal and local levels. Whilst there are some highly skilled managers in place, in general there is a dearth of appropriately skilled staff. Given the choice, doctors may immerse themselves in never ending clinical responsibilities in order to escape from the more fraught task of managing services.

Yet management is rarely taught in medical undergraduate schools,

---

Box 4.5

ASSOCIATION OF SWISS MEDICAL DOCTORS

The vast majority of Swiss medical professionals is organized in a private association called FMH (Foederatio Medicorum Helveticorum). This professional organization started in 1932 and had its origins in various medical societies, of which the earliest was founded in 1867. In 1991 almost 25,000 physicians (more than 95 per cent of all physicians in Switzerland) were in this organization. The main tasks of the organization are:

- Representing the interests of the medical profession including the pricing policy for medical practitioners and specialists.
- Determining the content of training programmes for specialists and the awarding of specialist degrees.
- Editing a weekly journal, which includes, besides professional articles, the prime advertisement forum for medical job opportunities in Switzerland.
- An arbitration committee which can advise patients on liability cases.
- Voluntary quality control in some specialities, such as laboratory medicine.

The association is organized in regions and related to specialities. The association is self-financed and receives no external funding. Most of the paramedical professions, like nurses or midwives, are controlled by the Swiss Red Cross, which also has a nongovernmental status. Only a few technical professions, like X-ray assistants, are governed by federal legislation.

Source: Verbindung der Schweizer Ärzte (1991)

---

and long term management development is unusual apart from in donor-led management strengthening projects. Due to the expectations of health professionals and administrators it is often difficult to reconcile their needs and expectations and those of the users (Jeannée and Lorenz 1991).

Possible solutions

Health management in most countries is not viewed as a specific profession. Whilst a public health background is a good basis for a health service manager, it is not enough. Innovative and active 'movers' are needed. Managers need to understand what people want; what health services are effective at providing; what services they have, and how they can be changed to make them more efficient and effective. These people will be assisted by appropriate training in management theory; and training in useful tools, including needs assessment, management by objectives, resource management, human resource development and epidemiology. But good managers are also not enough. The managerial environment in which they work has to be structured so that managers can be effective. This will require:

- giving them appropriate responsibility and authority to act as managers in human and financial resource management;
- a good working environment with adequate equipment and a minimum of material and financial resources to work with;

Box 4.6

ACCREDITATION SCHEMES IN MEXICO

In Mexico the National Secretary of Health has promoted the implementation of a voluntary accreditation system for hospitals from the private and public sector. They initiated the process by holding two national conferences of consensus with the involvement of all interested parties who were consulted about the feasibility of establishing a process of voluntary accreditation for hospitals in Mexico. They were also consulted about the format and attributions that such a process should take. The conferences involved more than 60 people representing all the major private hospitals in Mexico, as well as representatives of all the public institutions in Mexico that manage hospitals as part of the health services that they provide. Decentralized public hospitals were also represented as well as a number of associations of public and private hospitals and major medical associations such as the National Academy of Medicine, the Mexican Association of Hospitals, the Mexican Society for Quality of Health care etc.

As a result of such conferences there was general agreement that the accreditation should be done by an autonomous body or organization that has the following characteristics: autonomous, nongovernmental, national, representative of all sectors and health institutions, nonprofit, with voluntary affiliation, self-sufficient in budgetary terms. The institutions that should be represented in such a mixed organization were identified having ten representatives from the public sector, a representation of the private sector (in this case hospitals) and five representatives of the social sector.

The financial mechanisms were also defined; thus the main contribution to the organization should come from the fees that will be paid by the hospitals that apply to be evaluated for accreditation; also, a fee will be established for all the members of the organization in order to start the process. Donations from interested organizations were identified as a third possible source of financial support.

The process for accreditation in Mexico under this configuration of voluntary accreditation has just started, but it was perceived by all the participants as the best alternative to standardize the quality of care provided by all hospitals in Mexico. There are no punitive measures attached to this process. The only outcome is the gain and value added by the fact of being an accredited hospital.

- staff that have adequate pay;
- functional and constructive monitoring;
- access to continuous training and advice; and
- involvement of health workers in decision making.

These changes will require more effective decentralization: central agencies may profess commitment to a process of decentralization, but frequently resources and power remain centrally controlled. Decentralization, with a team approach to management, is sometimes successful. In Dar es Salaam, district health managers are meeting on a weekly basis to discuss city health issues. District health management teams also meet on a regular basis. This has made the decision making processes more transparent. Furthermore, districts have a centrally allocated budget, which they can administer on the basis of locally established budgets. This has led to an increased awareness of responsibility of the persons in charge. Locally generated revenue, for example from ambulance services, is also used locally. Uniforms, a need expressed by the health workers, could be bought with local funds. These measures have increased the effectiveness of the system in spite of insufficient salaries and poor career prospects (Dar es Salaam Urban Health Project 1992).

THE PROCESS OF CHANGE

Health care is highly political. Poor performance of health services and unaffordable costs are reasons for dissatisfaction and have considerable potential for social unrest. Ill health is a risk to us all, and medical technology appears to offer hope of cure. Faith in technology on an individual basis, coupled with overprovision of care (especially by private providers), creates a large demand for complex care that costs a lot and may be of unproven effectiveness. Indeed, whilst high technology care is almost always inaccessible to most people in less developed countries, this does not stop people hoping that when they need it they will have access to it. Thus politicians who are supportive of highly visible complex medical care are more likely to catch people's votes. Doctors too are guilty of providing care of unknown effectiveness.

Improving health care in cities will require *political will* to change. This requires a commitment to good quality care of proven effectiveness; strong managerial control over professional self-interest; and commitment to equitable distribution of resources, ensuring that poorer (and therefore sicker) groups receive a basic minimum package of effective care.

In practical terms this requires *a shift in power* so that planners and managers have authority over clinicians in resource allocation; and *structural change* towards decentralization of the responsibility for various aspects of health care. Smaller units need to control their own resources, and to be directly accountable to senior managers for their outputs and improving the quality and efficiency of the care they provide.

Due to global changes there is increasing pressure for *democratizing public services*, to make them of better quality, more efficient and responsive to the needs of the public they serve. This could form the basis of making something more tangible out of the sometimes vague concept of community participation. Whilst service content, form and quality are often determined by professionals, it is time to make services more accountable to the users, and thus ensure that they take into account the views, perceptions and expectations of the urban population served.

REFERENCES

Anon (1993) White Elephants about Town *Lancet*, 341, pp1563–1564

Ashton, J (1993) Reference Health Centres (correspondence) *Lancet*, 342, pp372–373

Astagneau, P Lang, T Delarocque, E Jeanée, E and Salem, G (1992) Arterial Hypertension in Urban Africa: an Epidemiological Study on a Representative Sample of Dakar Inhabitants in Senegal *Journal of Hyptertension*, 10, pp1095–1101

Bennett, S (1992) Promoting the Private Sector: a Review of Developing Country Trends *Health Policy and Planning*, 7, pp97–110

Bennett, S Dakpallah, G Garner, P Gilson, L Nittayaramphong, S and Zwi, A (1994) Carrot and Stick: State Mechanisms to Influence Private Provider Behaviour *Health Policy and Planning*, 9, pp1–13

Child, J (1984) *Organization: a Guide to the Problems and Practice* Harper and Row, London

Dar es Salaam Urban Health Project (1992) Internal Document Swiss Tropical Institute, Basel, Switzerland

Ebrahim, G Ranken, J (eds) (1988) *Primary Health Care: Reorienting Organizational Support* MacMillan, London

Garner, P and Thaver, I (1993) Urban Slums and Primary Health Services *British Medical Journal*, 306, pp667–668

Gilson, L Kilima, P and Tanner, M Local Government Decentralization and the Health Sector in Tanzania *Journal of Public Administration and Development* (in press)

Gonzàlez, L Mora, J and Aponte, J (1992) *Advanced Units for Comprehensive Health Care: Description of the General Model* Instituto Nacional de Salud Pública (Secretaria de Salud del Gobierno de Veracruz), mimeo, pp1–19

Gordon, J Mondy, R Sharplin, A and Premeaux, S (1990) *Management and Organizational Behaviour* Allyn and Bacon, Boston

Holdsworth, G Garner, P Harpham, T and Mosala, N (1994) Crowded Outpatient Departments in City Hospitals of Developing Countries: a Case Study from Lesotho *International Journal of Health Planning and Management*, 8 (4), pp315–324

Hülsebusch, B (1993) Ärzteskandal in Italien: 'Professoren' legen Patienten aufs Kreuz *Badische Zeitung*, 18, p5

Jeaneé, E and Lorenz, N (1991) Projet Pikine: 15 ans d'expérience, un modèle? *Afrique Médecine et Santé*, 61, pp39–40

Kanji (personal communication)

Kanji, N Kilima, P Lorenz, N and Garner, P Primary Health Care in Dar es Salaam: a Comparison of Government and Voluntary Health Services *Health Policy and Planning* (in press)

King, M (1966) *Medical Care in Developing Countries* Oxford University Press, Nairobi

Klein, R (1993) Dimensions of Rationing: Who Should Do What? *British Medical Journal*, 307, pp309–311

Lee, K and Mills, A (1982) *Policy-making and Planning in the Health Sector* Croom Helm, Beckenham

McKeown, T (1979) *The Role of Medicine* Blackwell, Oxford

Mills, A (1990a) The Economics of Hospitals in Developing Countries Part 1: Expenditure Patterns *Health Policy and Planning*, 5, pp107–117

Mills, A (1990b) The Economics of Hospitals in Developing Countries Part 2: Costs and Sources of Income *Health Policy and Planning*, 5, pp203–218

Mills, A Vaughan, J Smith, D and Tabibzadeh, I (1990) *Health System Decentralization: Concepts, Issues and Country Experiences* World Health Organization, Geneva

Normand, C (1991) Economics, Health and the Economics of Health *British Medical Journal*, 303, pp1572–1577

Pepperall, J and Garner, P (1992) *The Maseru Hospital and Health Centre Outpatient Care Study: Research Findings and Implications*. Report from the London School of Hygiene and Tropical Medicine, Ministry of Health Lesotho, and Queen Elizabeth II Hospital Maseru (mimeo), pp1–68.

Segall, M (1991) Health Sector Planning Led by Management of Recurrent Expenditure: an Agenda for Action Based Research *International Journal of Health Planning and Management*, 6, pp37–75

Shepard, D Walsh, J Munar, W Rose, L Guerrero, R Cruz, L Reyes, G Orsolani, G and Solarte, C (1993) Cost-effectiveness of Ambulatory Surgery in Cali, Colombia *Health Policy and Planning*, pp136–142

Verbindung der Schweizer Ärzte (1991) *Vademecum für den Schweizer Arzt* Ott Verlag, Bem 5, Auglage

World Bank (1993) *World Development Report 1993: Investing in Health* Oxford University Press, Washington

World Health Organization (1991) Improving Urban Health Systems *World Health Statistics Quarterly*, 44, pp234–240

World Health Organization (1992) The Role of Health Centres in the Development of Urban Health Systems *WHO Technical Report Series* no. 827, pp1–38

5

Research on Urban Health –
the Priorities and Approaches

John R Seager

INTRODUCTION

U rban health research in developing countries is not a new discipline but it is time for some new approaches. Much of the early urban health research was dominated by descriptive epidemiological approaches but, in order to place health risks in a sociocultural context, there is a need to supplement the research with relevant sociological and anthropological studies. Increasingly, the need for an even wider interdisciplinary approach is being recognised and the research team should then include demographers, urban planners, engineers and community development specialists. Rather than describing specific methodology, most of which can be found in general epidemiology and human sciences textbooks, this chapter aims to highlight some of the peculiarities and pitfalls of urban health research. Examples from recent research are used to illustrate some of these points.

Initially it is useful to consider what research is and how it differs from evaluation. The two terms are sometimes confused, especially in service delivery where research may not be considered a 'legitimate' function whereas evaluation is seen as having a more immediate value and can therefore be more easily justified. In reality, research and evaluation are the two ends of a continuum and the difference is determined largely by what motivates the question. In the case of fundamental research, the question may be motivated by nothing more than curiosity or, in the somewhat ostentatious terms of the academic, 'the quest for knowledge'. In a purely academic environment this may be sufficient reason for doing research but is unlikely to be acceptable to a city health official or an urban community. At the other end of the continuum is evaluation which can only be done once some kind of intervention is in place to be evaluated. The question is then motivated by a concern to know how well something is working, usually in terms of health outcomes and sometimes in terms of cost benefits. A critical factor, however, which is often overlooked in the purely epidemiological or financial assessment, is the quality of life, and this can only be properly assessed by the interdisciplinary approach.

Looking at the extremes of the continuum is likely to result in howls of protest from proponents of either side since few researchers or evaluators totally exclude the other approach. The important point is that urban health research may be driven by curiosity but the topic of investigation must be something which is amenable to intervention (or for which there is at least a workable hypothesis for intervention). Similarly, evaluation must not become destructive criticism (which is often how it is perceived by overworked service providers) but must identify problems which can be further investigated by research and for which solutions can be found.

Given that there is potential for the improvement of existing urban health initiatives by evaluation and research, it becomes obvious that urban health research must not be an independent activity but one that is closely linked to the social sector in general and the health sector in particular. Failure to develop this close link has, in the past, resulted in research which is often merely descriptive and has little relevance to the practical needs of service providers or the population. Urban health research which was either not sufficiently relevant to actual needs or was inadequately explained to the potential end user has contributed to difficulties in attracting the necessary funding for new research.

In addition, economic recession exacerbates the problem, and research tends to be seen as a luxury which can be deferred until the economic situation improves. In developing countries, economic constraints make this an almost permanent situation so research often receives a low priority. However, it is when money and resources are in short supply that research into how to make the best use of limited resources becomes critical. Conducting research on the right issues in the right way should make a difference to both the health of urban populations and their general quality of life.

URBAN HEALTH RESEARCH IN DEVELOPING COUNTRIES

At the turn of the century, more than half the world's population will be living in cities. This will have a profound effect on global health and consequently make new demands on public health research. The developing countries are the least urbanized yet the urban population of the developing world already exceeds that of Europe, America and Japan combined (World Health Organization 1993).

Urban health research faces many special problems and, despite the attempts to prevent rapid urbanization which have been made in many countries, urban growth seems to be inevitable. Typically, a large proportion of the urban population of developing countries lives in underserviced, poor quality housing with inadequate access to health care. But, as Dr Hiroshi Nakajima, Director-General of the World Health Organization, pointed out to the 44th World Health Assembly in 1991 (see the chapter by Goldstein et al), urbanization is not necessarily bad in itself.

It becomes a problem when the rate of growth of the urban population exceeds the capacity of the infrastructure to absorb and support it. There is an urgent need to conduct research into urban health which will provide policy guidelines to allow healthy development of cities.

Life in the urban environment should offer numerous advantages such as better access to education, employment, sustainable food supplies and health care. Urban health research therefore has the responsibility to quantify the impact of urbanization on health; to identify current and likely future risk factors for poor health influenced by urbanization; to design and test appropriate interventions and to provide information which will allow policy makers, service providers and the community to make informed decisions about health within the urban environment.

Another good reason for giving urban health research high priority is that health is a *contributory* factor to development and not merely a *consequence* of development (Commission on Health Research for Development 1990). The public health movement began during the 19th century when, with the progress of the industrial revolution, employers realized that a healthy workforce was essential to better productivity. Later, an accepted definition of public health included 'promoting health and efficiency' (Winslow 1920). The same principle applies to the efficiency or productivity of countries and, when correctly managed or governed, high productivity of a country results from the good health of its population.

A critical issue for urban health research is the enigma that a very large proportion of morbidity and mortality in the developing world is the result of preventable disease. These diseases are usually poverty related and can be prevented by relatively simple interventions such as vaccination or can be 'engineered' out of the environment. Infectious diseases such as gastroenteritis and measles are major causes of death in infants, yet both are preventable. Poor sanitation and inadequate water supplies are the major determinants of gastroenteritis and the coverage of measles vaccination is too low to prevent measles epidemics in overcrowded peri-urban areas. These diseases have, for many years, been well controlled in the developed world but remain a serious problem in the developing world.

As urbanization proceeds, urban populations in developing countries also begin to experience more of the diseases of affluence which are predominantly chronic diseases (Jamison et al 1993). The most marked increases are in ischaemic heart disease and lung cancer associated with changes in lifestyle, changes in diet and the acquisition of habits such as smoking and drinking alcohol. The lifestyle changes are frequently related to advertising and new social pressures. This epidemiological transition from 'old' to 'new' disease patterns or, in the case of the developing world, the 'epidemiological trap' producing the worst of both worlds is a major challenge to urban health research.

SETTING PRIORITIES FOR RESEARCH

Priority setting in urban health research is a thorny issue but must be carefully considered when resources are limited as in most developing countries. Interviews with several hundred health and related

---

Box 5.1

CRITERIA INFLUENCING PRIORITY SETTING FOR PUBLIC HEALTH RESEARCH

1. *Health problem focus (prioritize problems)*
   - Magnitude of the health problem
     – Numbers involved
     – Is the health problem communicable?
   - Impact/seriousness
     – Financial
     – Human suffering
     – Benefit of health improvement
   - Vulnerability to management
     – Can the problem be prevented?
     – Is it amenable to remediation?
     – Cost of intervention
   - Extent of community concern

2. *Population focus (prioritize people)*
   - Do certain populations experience greater morbidity/mortality?
   - What is age, gender, race, geographic distribution?
   - Have the needs of certain groups or areas been neglected?

3. *Health service focus (prioritize problems in services)*
   - Magnitude of the problem
   - Impact/seriousness
   - Vulnerability to management
   - Extent of community concern
   - Extent of provider concern

4. *Researcher focus (prioritize by researcher variables)*
   - Interests of researchers/intellectual challenge
   - Available skills of the research community
   - Scientific feasibility
   - Affordability of the research
   - Availability of funding from other sources
   - Need for further research on this topic
   - Balance of competing protocols

5. *General issues*
   - Responsive to local and regional differences
   - Time focus of the research
     – Estimated time until payoff
     – Prospective versus retrospective focus
     – Pre- versus post-transitional focus
   - Social/ethical implications of addressing problem
   - Significance for training/capacity development

Source: Yach et al (1991)

---

professionals in South Africa led Yach et al (1991) to identify five areas which influence priority setting (Box 5.1).

These five areas each reflect different foci for the priority setting

Box 5.2

A DECISION MAKING HIERARCHY FOR PUBLIC HEALTH INTERVENTIONS

1. Diseases which are easily preventable should take precedence over those which are difficult to prevent.
2. Diseases which have a high cost of treatment should take precedence over diseases which have low treatment costs.
3. Diseases which are life threatening, disabling or of long duration should take precedence over diseases which are of a passing nature.
4. Diseases which occur with a high prevalence/incidence/mortality rate should take precedence over those which occur at a low rate.
5. Communicable diseases should take precedence over noncommunicable diseases.

Source: Bradshaw et al 1988

process ie whether the focus is on the health problem itself; the people it affects; the impact these people have on the health services; the research environment; or general issues. An important point which, in this analysis, appears near the end of the list, should not be overlooked, and that is the social and ethical implications of addressing the problem. Public opinion can be an important factor when deciding on research priorities and it may be necessary to address issues of public concern before other less obvious, yet significant, health problems. Clearly the background of the individual deciding priorities will influence his or her perception so it is advisable to consult widely before taking decisions. To this end, the Delphi approach (Dalkey 1969), which has as one of its principles anonymous expression of ideas, may be a useful method for achieving consensus (Saayman et al 1991).

Another approach was taken by Bradshaw et al (1988) who suggested a set of decision making rules which can be used in a mathematical hierarchy (Box 5.2). Friedman (1991) took a similar approach (Box 5.3) to arrive at a formula for determining health care priorities which could also apply to urban health research.

These methods have the appeal of a semi-quantitative approach, but where sub-groups of the population, such as the poor, experience disproportionately high burdens of ill health this in itself may be sufficient reason to give these groups high priority for research (Feachem et al 1989). *The World Development Report* for *1993: Investing in Health* (World Bank 1993) provides a comprehensive overview of global public health priorities. In practice, a combination of subjective methods, based on local knowledge, and objective methods, drawing on general models, needs to be used to arrive at an urban health research agenda which will meet the needs of a country and all its urban people.

Box 5.3

DETERMINING PRIORITIES FOR URBAN HEALTH RESEARCH

Magnitude: (based on prevalence statistics from a field study)
1.   Acute morbidity (AM)
2.   Chronic morbidity (CM)
3.   Mortality (MO)

Impact/seriousness: (based on statistics derived from a Community Medical Ward)
1.   Incidence of ICD groups requiring admission (IN)
2.   Case fatality (CF)

Vulnerability to management: (arbitrary scoring)
1.   Prevention (PV)
2.   Treatment (TR)

Concern: (based on views expressed during community survey)
1.   Problems identified by the community (PB)
2.   Priorities identified by community (PR)

Cost: (based on average days of hospital stay for each ICD group)
1.   Cost expressed in terms of patient days (CS)

Using the following mathematical function, a value for priority is calculated for each ICD group:

$$\text{Priority} = \text{Magnitude} \times \text{Impact} \times \text{Vulnerability} \times \text{Concern} \times \text{Cost}$$
$$= (AM \times CM \times MO) \times (IN \times CF) \times (PV \times TR) \times (PB \times PR) \times CS$$

Source: Adapted from Friedman 1991

A STRATEGY FOR RESEARCH ON URBAN HEALTH

Given scarce resources, the first priority for any developing country's research programme will be to look at problems which are specific to that particular country. The Commission on Health Research for Development (1990) stated that 'every country, no matter how poor, must carry out this type of research to make the best use of its limited resources'. The Commission referred to this core of research as Essential National Health Research (ENHR). The first research objective then becomes to select priority health problems which have a major impact on the country's health system; once these problems have been successfully addressed, it will be easier to mobilize public support, and consequently the policy makers, to make further improvements in the health sector.

One of the many advantages of the ENHR strategy is that the research addresses real priorities for the country concerned and topics are put in context with regard to national priorities in health. There is a very real risk that research carried out by international aid agencies may be meeting a global agenda (which may well have its merits) but does not really address the priorities for the country where the research is done. There is, however, a need for developing countries to join some global research projects on broader issues for which basic knowledge is still lacking, and where collaborative projects are probably the best way to achieve results which can be applied in a wide range of settings.

The common health problems affecting the urban population in developing countries are often closely linked to environmental factors, socioeconomic conditions and of course the specific health risks of the country concerned (see the chapter by Tanner and Harpham). These types of problems invariably require input from public health researchers, health service providers, social scientists, environmental consultants, water and sanitation specialists, educationalists and economists. Interdisciplinary teams which include such a wide range of participants are rare but are probably the key to successful research and effective implementation of the results.

Given the size of the task and the complex teams required to carry out effective urban health research, many researchers may feel that this type of work is beyond their scope, but collaborative programmes can provide the necessary skills. Faced with such a task in South Africa, a small group of epidemiologists began a networking process in 1988 and since then have developed a research programme which has facilitated over 50 projects running in most major urban centres in the country. The strategy followed was first to engage with those university departments which had the essential epidemiology research skills (community health departments) and then to recruit additional partners once a few successful projects had been publicized.

A critical factor was securing some initial funding which could be rapidly made available for new projects in what was regarded as a high priority research area. Some 'venture funding' was made available in order to get projects off the ground and, for the first time, funds were provided to assist potential collaborators with preparing proposals. In order to achieve the desired results, the small core of epidemiologists usually worked very closely with potential collaborators and, in most cases, successful protocols were prepared and the studies subsequently carried out. Some of these projects were funded from the same initial source and others produced sufficiently substantial proposals for other agencies to be willing to fund the research.

As this pioneering work progressed, a conscious effort was made to publicize the initial results as quickly as possible. This was done via a quarterly *Urbanization and Health Newsletter* which was distributed free of charge. The aim of this newsletter was twofold: firstly it publicized initial findings long before formal publications could be produced; secondly it informed other researchers, via review articles and interviews with public health specialists, of the importance and potential of urban health research. The *Newsletter* has become a popular source of current research information and has a circulation of nearly 600 of which 40 are to other African countries and 90 to countries around the world. The rapid release of pre-publication results contributes to the successful development and improvement of other current projects. The advantages of this type of communication network are considerable and with increasing electronic communication, even in the poorer countries, more information exchange should be encouraged. There is too much work waiting to be done for researchers to keep their results as closely guarded secrets and free information exchange will tend to reduce the chance of unnecessary duplication. The researchers also benefit from the newsletter format in that the articles can be written relatively quickly, summarizing major findings, without jeopardizing subsequent formal publication. One risk with this approach is that incomplete studies may produce erroneous results so the editorial policy of such publications must ensure that work publicized is methodologically sound and that the often preliminary nature of the findings is clearly stated.

METHODOLOGICAL ISSUES

Defining the urban area

Various definitions of what is 'urban' have been used and, in general, it is necessary to clearly define both the area and the population under study for each specific project. Graaf (1987) proposed a number of criteria for defining the urban environment which include the type of administration present, population density, economic aspects such as whether income is agricultural or industrial, and level of access to basic services. Census data often define urban as any area which falls under some form of local government authority but this criterion will often exclude large sectors of the population living on the urban fringe in informal settlements.

Another simple but quite useful definition can be to use distance from the city centre to define areas for making intra-urban comparisons. In a small city in Transkei, Byarugaba (1991) classified the zone up to five km from the city centre as urban, five–ten km as peri-urban and rural for all locations/settlements further than ten km from the city centre. Clearly in megacities these distances could be much greater but for comparative purposes distance defined zones of a metropolitan area can be a useful approach. Care should be exercised in making certain of the type of settlement being studied since, in some situations, settlements at great distances from major cities may have an almost entirely urban economy. This would be the case of 'dormitory towns' which offer low cost housing for either daily or even annual migrants to the city.

Measuring urbanization

If exposure to the urban environment is a risk factor for a health problem being investigated, some measure of 'urban exposure' is necessary. One of the simplest and probably most effective ways of measuring urban exposure is to look at the period of residence in the urban environment. Comparisons between recent arrivals (say less than three years), those who have grown up in the urban environment (say 10–15 years) and those who have lived in an urban environment for their entire lives will provide useful data. In many developing countries, however, settlement in the urban environment is not a simple one way migration process, so urban exposure can only properly be investigated by obtaining a detailed migration history. A common misconception is that all peri-urban squatters are recent arrivals from the rural areas but there is also a large proportion of these people who represent the overflow from overcrowded formal urban settlements. Similarly, some residents of urban areas may return to the rural areas for prolonged periods eg for schooling, or rural people become temporary urban residents in order to obtain health care eg for childbirth.

As mentioned previously, disease patterns change with urban exposure and patterns of risk factors for conditions such as cardiovascular disease may be sufficiently closely related to urbanization to be used as a proxy for urbanization (K Steyn, personal communication). Our knowledge of these processes is still relatively limited but such indicators could prove useful in the future.

Routine data versus specialized surveys

A common failing of routinely available health data is that the statistics are combined at each higher level of reporting in a way that tends to lose a great deal of detail. It is vitally important, however, to disaggregate health data for large metropolitan areas in order to highlight intra-urban health differentials. Many of the larger cities in the world can boast an overall health status which is extremely good but if one looks at the health of the urban poor, even in the most developed countries, key health indicators may be three or four times worse than those of the most affluent areas (Bradley et al 1992, Satterthwaite 1993). The official reports of Medical Officers of Health usually show the city to be 'healthier' than the rural areas but the real situation is often the reverse, especially as the poorest of the poor are frequently 'unofficial' residents of the city and may have been completely excluded from the routine health statistics.

Study designs – quantitative and qualitative methods

Urban health research studies fall into three broad categories:

1. Quantitative approaches based on classical epidemiological descriptive and analytical methods and/or sociological studies with structured or semi-structured interviews.
2. Qualitative approaches which use anthropological methods such as observation, focus group discussions and in-depth interviews.
3. Combinations of 1 and 2. These are often used in health systems research, action research and community based action research ('recherche populaire' as it is widely known in Francophone Africa).

In order to describe the health status of urban communities, quantitative cross-sectional studies, often using a questionnaire as the main survey instrument, have been widely used. This approach gathers a great deal of information relatively quickly but is methodologically weak in that it merely describes the situation at a point in time. More sophisticated techniques are required if risk factors are to be properly investigated. Longitudinal studies which investigate the impact of urban exposure on health over prolonged periods are the ideal (Fonn et al 1991) but invariably these studies are extremely costly and often beyond the financial means of developing countries. Blum and Feachem (1983) reviewed a large number of studies on the benefits of water and sanitation and found serious methodological limitations in most studies. They proposed wider use of case-control study designs which, because of smaller sample sizes, invariably reduce cost, and the case-control methodology ensures sufficient statistical power to properly identify risk factors.

Quantitative methodology has its limitations and there is growing support for supplementing it with qualitative methods. Recent research (Cooper et al 1990) has highlighted the limitations of questionnaire surveys in getting to the real issues at community level. This study supplemented questionnaires with in-depth interviews and focus group discussions. In this method, small groups of eight to ten similar subjects, who may be community representatives, health service providers or even developers, are encouraged to discuss issues pertinent to the health of the population. These discussions are deliberately kept informal with a few questions being used to focus the discussion on specific issues but allowing the participants freedom to discuss as they please.

In most studies where qualitative methods are used they inform the quantitative study which follows by providing a better understanding of the community under investigation. However, informal discussions often raise issues which are simply not detected in quantitative methods. There is a common tendency for poorly educated respondents to formal questionnaires to provide answers which they feel are 'correct' or will please the researchers. This problem can largely be overcome by using informal discussions with an observer taking notes of matters raised. A typical example of information which is hard to elicit is the use of traditional healers as a feature of health service utilization. Questionnaire surveys rarely obtain much information on traditional practices because of an apparent reluctance to discuss alternative health care with researchers who are often associated with conventional health services.

The natural follow on from the focus group approach is to involve the community members themselves in the research process in what is known as participatory research. Whilst community members may lack the necessary skills to carry out their own research, they can certainly be involved in the planning of the study and very often provide personnel for fieldwork and data cleaning. The essence of participatory research is that research ends up being done *with* communities rather than *on* communities. This approach is important because community participation can lead to a better understanding of the issues facing the community and consequently the researchers. Health is rarely the first priority on a community's agenda but the provision of basic services such as water, sanitation and waste removal is usually seen as a high priority (Matthews et al 1991), so these interventions can be used as a vehicle for other health initiatives (see Figure 5.1). This type of information is critical in the design of both the research project and health interventions as, without meeting the perceived community needs, as well as the legitimate priority health issues, the intervention phase of any research is likely to fail.

Sampling informal settlements

Since much of the developing world's urban areas comprise informal settlements and both health services and surveillance systems are often inadequate (Botha and Bradshaw 1985), particularly in the peri-urban areas, there is often insufficient baseline data to allow conventional sampling strategies. Maps and population statistics are the stock in trade tools of the

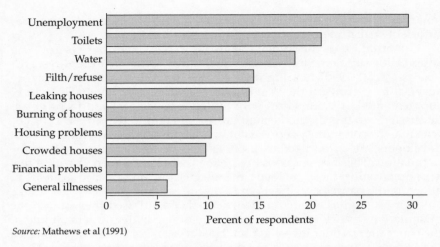

Source: Mathews et al (1991)

Figure 5.1 *Public health related problems as perceived by residents of an informal settlement (Khayelitsha, Cape Town)*

epidemiologist when beginning any research project but these are often unavailable or inaccurate. Typically a town plan may show an area officially designated for informal settlement (for example self-build housing projects) with spaces for parks, soccer fields and schools but the situation on the ground is quite different. As soon as land is cleared and some amenities are provided, people move in and 'squat' on all available land. Given a situation where settlements are either not mapped or the available maps are inaccurate, and population statistics are often little better than educated guesses, alternative methodologies have to be considered.

Making maps specifically for research purposes is one strategy but is not always successful. Mapping small rural settlements is relatively easy but the informal peri-urban sprawl of most developing country cities is very difficult to map. Added to this is the problem of rapid growth in these settlements which makes maps obsolete within a matter of months. Aerial photographs can be useful for mapping but are subject to errors in that it is often impossible to distinguish between houses and shops or storerooms. Photographs will always need to be supplemented by sample surveys to link population estimates to physical structures.

Many compromises will have to be made when sampling in these communities and it is often necessary for the researcher to spend much more time than expected in the field. Variations on simple stratified random sampling are often the only practical solution. Whilst the purist may feel that such samples may not produce sufficiently generalizable results, it is inappropriate to carry out sampling with a higher degree of precision than is warranted by the survey instruments. In other words, questionnaires on urban health problems are unlikely to achieve precision much better than 80 per cent so there is little point in sampling to a precision of 95 per cent. This is not to say that obtaining the most representative sample possible should be ignored but practical considerations almost invariably mean that conventional sample size determinations have to be modified.

RECENT RESEARCH RESULTS

Having defined the area of study ie the urban environment in a particular investigation, we need to consider what are the most important issues for investigation. The priority setting methods described above will give assistance in determining research needs but there are three main categories of health problems which are associated with urbanization (Tabibzadeh et al 1989). These are health problems related to poverty; diseases associated with industrialization; and health problems resulting from political and social instability. The examples that follow are by no means exhaustive but serve to illustrate the sorts of issues which urban health research should explore.

Poverty related diseases

Of the poverty related diseases, those which can be prevented by cheap and effective vaccines, yet still kill thousands of infants each year, are perhaps among the most frustrating. Measles is one example and measles vaccination coverage among children under two years of age is related to home delivery, having been born outside the urban setting and length of stay in the city (Coetzee et al 1991a, Coetzee et al 1991b). Children born in rural areas are generally less likely to have been vaccinated than those born in the urban area (Table 5.1) but a critical finding is that new arrivals to the urban area are always occurring and warrant special attention (Berry et al 1991) if the effects of vaccination campaigns are to be sustained. A number of additional obstacles such as distance from health facilities, economic and cultural barriers, and inconvenient clinic hours all contribute to the problem.

Table 5.1 *Urbanization and vaccination coverage (children vaccinated at least once, Khayelitsha, Cape Town)*

	Before vaccination campaign	3 weeks after campaign	6 months after campaign
Place of birth			
Urban	62%	78%	79%
Rural	51%	80%	54%
Period in urban area			
<6 months	32%	70%	53%
>6 months	50%	66%	73%
Odds ratio	2.17	0.83	2.44

Source: Berry et al (1991)

Quality of housing is closely linked to poverty and von Schirnding et al (1991a) demonstrated high housing related risks for diarrhoeal disease and acute respiratory infections (ARI) in South African children. Three housing factors are particularly related to health and safety: the first is overcrowding; the second is inadequate utility services, and particularly important here are potable water supplies, refuse and sewage disposal facilities; and the third is quality of dwelling and shelter.

Individual risk factors identified for diarrhoea included not having an inside tap or a flush toilet in the home, not owning a refuse receptacle, not being connected to an electricity supply, low household income, more than two people per room and less than standard five maternal education (von Schirnding et al 1991a). The most important interventions therefore, for reducing childhood infections, are better access to water and sanitation, general environmental health services and probably improvements in access to electricity (Table 5.2).

Provision of electricity can change living conditions dramatically so that there are many indirect health benefits. These range from moving away from biomass fuels, with consequent reduction in respiratory health problems, to better education standards due to availability of domestic lighting for homework. The impacts are not always straightforward, however, and studies have shown that even with electrification, economic factors often result in many residents continuing to use biomass fuels (Terblanche et al 1993) so that health risks in electrified homes may not be significantly better than nearby unelectrified ones.

Table 5.2 *Prioritizing interventions for diarrhoea in children <5 years of age*

Risk factor	Odds ratio	90 per cent confidence interval	Intervention priority
No inside tap	3.3	1.7–5.0	1
No inside WC	3.3	2.5–5.0	1
Do not own refuse receptacle	2.5	1.3–5.0	2
No electricity	2.5	1.4–5.0	2
Overcrowding (>2 people/room)	2.0	1.3–3.3	3

Source: Adapted from von Schirnding et al 1991a

Many of these results are neither particularly startling nor new: in fact the Dean of Johns Hopkins Medical School reached a similar conclusion in 1893 when he said 'sanitary improvements offered the best way of improving the lot of the poor short of a radical restructuring of society'. Unfortunately there is good evidence that policy makers usually demand local data on specific health risks before they are willing to take action. The urban health researchers' job then becomes to present the most important locally relevant information in a form which is accessible to the policy makers.

Diseases associated with industrialization

Environmental pollution is also a feature of urbanization and in many cities the poor experience the highest exposure levels. Urban planning needs to address the siting of residential areas and schools away from sources of pollution such as heavy industry and major highways and information which will contribute to refining existing air and water quality legislation is required (Terblanche et al 1991). Most air pollution studies have tended to focus on the outdoor environment but recent work has shown the importance of indoor air quality monitoring. Identifying risk factors is relatively easy but devising affordable interventions is the real challenge.

Attention must also be given to the impact of informal sector activities on environmental health. In most developing countries a large part of the economy is informal and is often outside the normal control of environmental and occupational health legislation (Barten et al 1993, Jamison et al 1993) yet many of these activities are in high risk occupations.

Health problems related to social and political instability

Urbanization is also associated with profound changes in lifestyle which can affect the mental health of new arrivals. During settlement, links between the urban and the rural areas remain strong and a proportion of people's time is spent oscillating between the two which creates increased stress and instability at individual, home and community levels. People often move from one urban area to another within large cities and may also lose contact with their established support networks. The result of this type of change can create stress which is often manifested as mental disorder, alcohol and other substance abuse, or violence.

Alcohol misuse is responsible for a large proportion of motor vehicle accidents and contributes to conditions such as cancer of the oesophagus, cirrhosis of the liver, pancreatitis and the risk of sexually transmitted diseases. A recent review of South African studies indicated that there is a consistent pattern of high risk drinking behaviour among certain age and ethnic groups. Table 5.3 shows very high rates of risky drinking (≥five beers/day or equivalent among black males and although the rates are lower for females there is a tendency for more risky drinking in informal settlements). Extremely high rates of 'binge' drinking (≥five drinks on at least one occasion in the past 14 days) have also been reported for Cape Town high school students. Adolescents are a particularly vulnerable group in the urban environment and research is required to make sure they are not overlooked in health policy planning. Teenage pregnancy and street children are two outcomes which require further investigation.

IMPLEMENTATION OF RESEARCH RESULTS

Given that much of the ill health in urban areas of the developing world is caused by organisms and agents for which there are known preventive measures, it is clear that application of existing knowledge is an important part of the research process. This leads the urban health researcher into an area which has been the source of much debate (Lanes 1985, Rothman and Poole 1985), namely where to draw the line between research and implementation. Some argue that the researcher's job is merely to provide information on current and future health problems and to maintain a separation between the research and the implementation of the results since when the researcher becomes directly involved with implementation, the research itself may become compromised. Whilst this is a potentially

Table 5.3 *Alcohol misuse*

Sample site	Group	Gender	Risk drinking behaviour
1a Metropolitan areas	Black adults	M	37%
		F	19%
1b Informal areas	Black adults	M	37%
		F	25%
2 Cape Town	Adolescents	M	15–27%
		F	5–15 %

Source: 1 Rocha-Silva (1992) (risk criterion ≥5 beers/day or equivalent); 2 Flisher et al (1993) (risk criterion ≥5 drinks on at least one occasion in past 14 days)

serious issue, rigorous methodology and extensive peer review of both methods and results should prevent this type of bias from arising.

There is a wealth of evidence in the literature, much of which merely gathers dust on library shelves, to indicate that if researchers merely take their results to publication stage and no further, the information is rarely used. Operationalizing research results is a much neglected field. Current opinion is leaning towards the concept of Essential National Health Research which deals with multidisciplinary problems via an interdisciplinary approach to arrive at transdisciplinary solutions. This research must not only address priority health problems for the country concerned but also follow the process through to implementation and formal policy development (Commission on Health Research for Development 1990). In the developed world, a separation of research and action is often possible, with entire teams devoted to each small aspect of a health problem. In the developing countries, however, this is a luxury that can rarely be afforded, consequently the public health researcher should consider him or herself to be an implementer and in many cases an advocate for a healthier public policy.

Policy is usually determined using incomplete information from a large number of sources. Researchers must realize that their results will be only a small part of the policy makers' decision support system and the more accessible the information is, the more likely it is to be used. Thus, whereas a typical research report is probably 80 per cent results and 20 per cent recommendations (if that much), it would probably have a greater impact on policy if it were the other way around ie 20 per cent results and 80 per cent recommendations. Obviously the recommendations must be based on sufficient research data but the detail is irrelevant to the policy maker. In many cases it would be advisable for the researcher to go even further and suggest which of the recommendations is the most likely to succeed; in order to do this, the researcher will probably have to be involved in pilot interventions as well.

One way of facilitating the utilization of research is to bring researchers, service providers and policy makers closer together. They are usually in separate departments, sometimes under separate ministries and often in separate institutions. The urban health research specialist should have regular, formal contact with the implementers and in many cases should be part of the district health management team.

When assessing the impact of research on policy it is almost impossible to ascribe outcomes to specific activities. Implementation results from an accumulation of information which influences opinion until there is a critical mass which results in policy change. ENHR strives to achieve equity in health status for the entire population by addressing community needs. The days of a paternalistic approach to public health are numbered and the general population and the policy makers need to work together to achieve a healthy future. A degree of give and take on both sides is necessary to bring perceived needs and real priorities in line so that we can make progress towards the elusive goal of 'health for all'.

Considerable information about the determinants of ill health in urban areas has already been collected and researchers must be very careful not to continue with more and more descriptive studies without making use of existing knowledge. The ENHR strategy is designed to promote research that 'goes somewhere'. Priorities vary from country to country but there are more similarities than differences in the urban health problems of the developing countries.

CONCLUSION

This chapter has examined the challenge which urbanization poses for researchers. Urbanization is a complex phenomenon which affects a vast range of health issues so that prioritising research agendas becomes essential. The fundamental question should shift from 'What *can* we research?' to 'What *should* we research?' The latter question is answered using priority setting tools that help determine which health problems are of concern to society, have significant public health impact and are amenable to intervention.

In order to solve the complex health problems of urban society we need to foster interdisciplinary cooperation and to arrive at transdisciplinary solutions. The alternative, which we often see, is multidisciplinary research which arrives at different solutions from each discipline. The analogy in planning is where the housing department takes care of shelter, the transport department develops roads and the health department tries to repair the adverse health impacts of these developments. An integrated approach, in which all three departments work together for *one* solution is likely to be far better in the long run. This may sound like wishful thinking but is certainly the logical approach. In this regard, some of the developing countries which are currently undergoing radical reform (post-revolution or democratization) may, for once, have an advantage over the developed world namely that they are in a position to adopt radically different strategies.

The mechanisms for integrated health and development planning are still in their infancy, but the solution probably lies in a health systems approach which fully recognises the social and environmental setting of health problems. Ultimately, research methods need to be validated in different settings and assessed for their possible use in rapid assessment procedures which will be of practical use in monitoring and evaluating urban health development programmes.

REFERENCES

Barten, F van Naerssen, T Robotham, D et al (1993) *Health and Environment in the Cities in the Late Twentieth Century* Paper presented at the EPH/City '93 Conference, Antwerp

Berry, D J Yach, D Hennink, M H J (1991) An Evaluation of the National Measles Vaccination Campaign in the New Shanty Areas of Khayelitsha *South African Medical Journal*, 79: pp433–436

Blum, D Feachem, R D (1983) Measuring the Impact of Water Supply and Sanitation Investments on Diarrhoeal Diseases: Problems of Methodology *International Journal of Epidemiology*, 12: pp357–365

Botha, J L Bradshaw, D (1985) African Vital Statistics – A Black Hole? *South African Medical Journal*, 67: pp977–981

Bradley, D Stephens, C Harpham, T Cairncross, S (1992) *A Review of Environmental Health Impacts in Developing Country Cities* World Bank, Washington

Bradshaw, D Yach, D Fellingham, S A (1988) *Community-based Essential Health care Services in Southern Africa* Parrow: South African Medican Research Council

Byarugaba, J (1991) The Impact of Urbanization on the Health of Black Preschool Children in the Umtata district, Transkei, 1990 *South African Medical Journal*, 79: pp444–448

Coetzee, N Berry, D J Jacobs, M E (1991a) Measles Control in the Urbanising Environment *South African Medical Journal*, 79: pp440–444

Coetzee, N Yach, D Blignaut, R Fisher, SA (1991b) Measles Vaccination Coverage and Its Determinants in a Rapidly Growing Peri-urban Area *South African Medical Journal*, 78: pp733–737

Commission on Health Research for Development (1990) *Health Research: Essential Link to Equity and Development* New York: Oxford University Press

Cooper, D Pick, W M Myers, J E et al (1990) *A Study of the Effects of Urbanization on the Health of Women in Khayelitsha, Cape Town Working Paper Number 2: In-depth Interviews with Residents in Khayelistsha and Their Value in Informing and Complementing Quantitative Research* Cape Town: University of Cape Town

Dalkey, N C (1969) *The Delphi Method: An Experimental Study of Group Opinion*, Santa Monica, California: The Rand Corporation

Feachem, R G Graham, W J Timaeus, I M (1989) Identifying Health Problems and Health Research Priorities in Developing Countries *Journal of Tropical Medicine and Hygiene*, 91: pp133–191

Flisher, A J Ziervogel, C F Chalton, D O and Robertson, B A (1993) Risk Taking Behaviour of Cape Peninsula High School Students: IV Alcohol Use *South African Medical Journal*, 83: pp480–482

Fonn, S de Beer, M Kgamphe, S et al (1991) 'Birth to ten' – Pilot Studies to Test the Feasibility of a Birth Cohort Study Investigating the Effects of Urbanization in South Africa *South African Medical Journal*, 79: pp449–454

Friedman, I (1991) *Determining Priorities for Health care* In: Yach, D Martin, G McIntyre, J et al (1991) Changing Health in South Africa: Towards New Perspectives in Research Menlo Park, California: H J Kaiser Family Foundation

Graaf, J F de V (1987) The Present State of Urbanization in the South African Homelands Rethinking the Concepts and Predicting the Future *Development Southern Africa* 4: 46–66

Jamison, D T Mosley, W H Measham, A R Bobadilla, J L (1993) *Disease Control Priorities in Developing Countries* New York: Oxford University Press

Lanes, S (1985) Causal Inference Is Not a Matter of Science *American Journal of Epidemiology*, 122: pp550

Matthews, C van der Walt, H Hewitson, D Toms, I P Blignaut, R Yach, D (1991) Evaluation of a Peri-urban Community Health Worker Project in the Western Cape *South African Medical Journal*, 79: pp504–510

Rocha-Silva L (1992) *Alcohol/Drug-related Research in the RSA: Meeting the Challenge of the 1990s* Pretoria: Human Sciences Research Council

Rothman, K Poole, C (1985) Science and Policy Making *American Journal of Public Health*, 75: pp340–341

Saayman, G Phillips, H Kok, P (1991) *Urbanization Research in South Africa: Priorities for the 1990s* Pretoria: HSRC Publishers

Satterthwaite, D (1993) The Impact on Health of Urban Environments *Environment and Urbanization*, 5: pp87–111

Tabibzadeh, I Rossi-Espagnet, A Maxwell, R (1989) *Spotlight on the Cities: Improving Urban Health* Geneva: WHO

Terblanche, A P S Danford, I R Nel, C M E (1993) Household Energy Use in South Africa, Air Pollution and Human Health *Journal of Energy in Southern Africa*, 4: pp54–57

Terblanche, A P S Uys, L Nel, C M E (1991) Development and Application of Ambient Air Quality Standards *Clean Air*, 8: pp19–21

Von Schirnding, Y E R Yach, D Blignaut, R Mathews, C (1991a) Environmental Determinants of Acute Respiratory Symptoms and Diarrhoea in Young Coloured Children Living in Urban and Peri-urban Areas of South Africa *South African Medical Journal*, 79: pp457–461

Von Schirnding, Y E R Fuggle, R F Bradshaw, D (1991b) Factors Associated with Elevated Blood Lead Levels in Inner City Cape Town *South African Medical Journal*, 79: pp454–456

Winslow, C E A (1920) The Untilled Field of Public Health *Modern Medicine*, 2: p183

World Bank 1993 *World Development Report 1993: Investing in Health* New York: Oxford University Press

World Health Organization (1993) *The Urban Health Crisis: Strategies for Health for all in The Face of Rapid Urbanization: Report of the Technical Discussions at The Forty-Fourth World Health Assembly* Geneva: WHO

Yach, D Martin, G McIntyre, J et al (1991) *Changing Health in South Africa: Towards New Perspectives in Research* Menlo Park, California: H J Kaiser Family Foundation

6

Costing and Financing Urban Health and Environmental Services

Margaret Thomas and Barbara McPake

INTRODUCTION

Urban health related services have typically been characterized by domination of tertiary level hospital services and inequity of provision, both in terms of geographical concentration and socio-economic distribution of users. Reorientation towards primary care and meeting the needs of poorer and more inaccessible groups requires an activist role for city authorities in policy making. The need for information about finance is obvious. An important part of the policy maker's task is to influence and advise on the matching of the financing of services with major policy goals concerned with the distribution of services. Major discrepancies between policy goals and financing need to be analyzed. Strategic planning should address corrective actions such as reallocating public funds, providing incentives and disincentives in the private sector and seeking foreign aid.

The financing of services in the context of increasing cost of provision is a persistent concern of urban authorities. Before a city can consider what strategies to employ to improve health status, it is necessary to understand and assess present systems of financing and to be better informed of current trends. Lack of detailed information on existing service costs, revenues and expenditures in a city is a stumbling block to systematic planning of alternative strategies and how these might be financed. Cities therefore need to undertake periodic studies as an integral part of the planning process.

In this chapter an attempt is made to provide a framework for analyzing recurrent and capital expenditure in a city on health care, water and sanitation services and municipal environmental provision. The main providers of services and their sources of finance are identified and described, and the major issues arising from financing patterns discussed. The second section gives an overview of the range of sources involved and the issues presented by their diversity. The third section reviews public sources of finance and the fourth section, private. Section five considers insurance arrangements as a source of finance which is neither a pure public or private source. Section six considers the role of donor financing and section seven summarizes the main issues which have emerged from the preceding discussion and assesses the most important information gaps which should be addressed by an urban financing study. The chapter makes it clear that these information gaps are substantial in most cities. In the annex to this chapter, a proposed city study is outlined and the methods which could be used to collect relevant information are discussed

THE MIX OF PUBLIC AND PRIVATE FINANCE AND PROVISION IN THE CITY

Health, water and sanitation, and environmental services are rarely provided by one authority or agency in a city. Instead, the suppliers of services are many and exceptionally heterogeneous (Table 6.1) and there are multiple sources of funds. This heterogeneity often leads to overlap of responsibilities of local, state and national authorities (Bahl and Linn 1992). Besides a variety of public and quasi-public bodies (eg a social security system), providers and intermediaries can include: a strong private, modern medical care sector; large employers with health facilities; mission hospitals; several types of traditional practitioners; and newly established private contractors for supply of services like refuse collection and disposal. Table 6.1 shows the range of services provided in a city. These have characteristics which make their suitability for public or private financing and provision vary.

Using Table 6.1 for their own analysis, city authorities can identify the sources of funds, types of providers and their relative importance for the city. In many cities the most important source of finance for capital and recurrent expenditure is government (central and local). The flow of funds is not one way. Cities may already have made substantial contributions to government funds. Shanghai, for example, provides one-sixth of the national budget revenue of China (*Financial Times*, 4 March 1993). In recent years pressure on overall government resources has led to more funds coming from elsewhere. The other principal sources of finance are private payments, insurance schemes and donors.

Government financing includes expenditure at all levels of government, together with expenditure of public corporations or parastatals. Certain government activities such as providing and monitoring safe water and sanitation, air pollution control and preventive measures against infectious diseases, have public goods characteristics which make it difficult and inefficient to organize markets for their provision. They are eminently suited to be responsibilities of government and to be publicly financed.

Private financing of services can be direct or indirect. Direct payment includes payments made to a variety of health providers including private practitioners, mission and private hospitals and clinics, traditional healers and private pharmacists. Water supply and sewage collection are often financed via direct payments also. Indirect payment for services

Table 6.1 *Health, water and sanitation and environmental provision in a city: types of services and providers*

	Central Government					City govt & CBOs				
	Health ministry	Social security agency	Other agencies[a]	Public works & other agen	Regional, State & District Govt	Municipality	Smaller units	Ind & agric	PVOs miss & other	Private pracs, modern & traditional
1 Personal services (care of patients): Health facilities (hospitals, physicians' offices, etc):										
Outpatient:										
General (mostly treatment of ill patients)				N/A			N/A			
Specialist				N/A		N/A	N/A			
Inpatient:										
General (bed and nursing)				N/A			N/A			
Specialist services (deliveries, surgery etc)				N/A			N/A			
Urban PHC facilities				N/A						
2 Disease control programme, can include, singly or in combination:										
Vector control (eg spraying for malaria)		N/A	N/A	N/A			N/A		N/A	N/A
Population prophylaxis (eg mobile teams immunize or deparasitize slum areas		N/A	N/A	N/A			N/A		N/A	N/A
Environmental intervention (eg removing vegetation from stagnant canals/waterways to control schistosomiasis)		N/A	N/A	N/A			N/A		N/A	N/A

3 Other programmes:

Water

Sanitation:

Human waste disposal

General sewerage

Inspection (eg of food purveyors and processors)

Education and promotion of health and hygiene: through institutions (eg. schools)

through media (eg radio posters)

Control of pests and zoonotic diseases in domesticated animals

Control of pollution: air

water (eg from industrial sources)

Monitoring (eg for outbreaks of communicable diseases)

N/A	N/A	N/A		N/A	N/A	N/A	N/A
N/A	N/A	N/A			N/A	N/A	N/A
N/A	N/A	N/A			N/A	N/A	N/A
	N/A	N/A		N/A	N/A	N/A	N/A
N/A	N/A	N/A		N/A	N/A	N/A	N/A
N/A	N/A	N/A		N/A	N/A	N/A	N/A
N/A	N/A	N/A	N/A	N/A	N/A	N/A	N/A
N/A	N/A	N/A	N/A	N/A	N/A	N/A	N/A
N/A	N/A	N/A		N/A	N/A	N/A	N/A
N/A		N/A		N/A	N/A	N/A	N/A

Notes

Key: Reg = regional; Mun = municipality; CBOs = community based organizations; PVO = private voluntary organizations; Ind & agric = industry and agricultural enterprises parastatal and private; Priv pracs = private practitioners: modern and traditional; Miss = missionary; Agen = agencies N/A service not offered by this provider category.

a) defence ministries that provide health services for service persons; also police service, prisons and mental institutions that provide services for their employees and inmates.

Source: This table draws on the framework of one in de Ferranti, D (1985): *Paying for Health Services in Developing Countries.* Staff Working Paper 721, World Bank, Washington

covers items such as payment for health services by employers (usually large industrial or commercial complexes), and financing by nongovernment bodies of other activities. For example, a charitable community organization may be involved in pit latrine building. The last decade has seen moves towards an enhanced role for the private sector and for injection of capital from private sources (Bennett 1991, World Health Organization 1991, 1993). More resources may become available and private financing may substitute for government finance, relieving government of financial responsibility for some services such as the care of the elderly or refuse collection.

Insurance mainly covers health service provision, particularly curative, inpatient care (Mills 1983). Health insurance is a mixed source of finance as it usually draws contributions from employers and employees in the city and often also from government. Insurance schemes can be run by government or by private insurance companies. A third option is employer-based insurance. Employers or parastatals such as a national railway company may act as the third party collection agent with eligibility linked to employment status.

The financing role of donors is becoming increasingly important, especially in the poorest countries and in the most overcrowded cities. Multilateral and bilateral donors and, on a smaller scale, non-governmental agencies are all involved in offering funds to support projects and provide technical expertise.

The funding of services within a city therefore presents a complex picture. The fact that health care, water and sanitation services and environmental services rely on many and different sources of funds makes planning the most appropriate patterns of services overall more difficult. There can be duplication and overlap, and efficiency and equity become more difficult to define and pursue than in a system relying on one source. Nonetheless there are also advantages. A diversity of sources can often prove more robust in the context of a fluctuating economy. The following sections consider the issues arising from each source of finance in turn.

PUBLIC FINANCE AND PROVISION

National governments

A number of central government ministries are likely to be involved in city health related activities. These include the Ministry of Health, the Ministry of Water, the Ministry of Education and the Ministry of Local Government. Because government has the prime role in national policy making and strategic planning, frequently linked to proposals for three or five year development plans, it may often appear that government is the principal actor.

Information on expenditure by central government in a particular city is often difficult to disentangle from national accounts whereas information relating to local government activities and expenditure can often be analyzed more easily using city accounts.

Analysis of central government expenditure according to its distributional implications will often reveal substantial inequities. Indonesian data show that government subsidy often favours higher

Table 6.2 *Government and household health expenditure – all Indonesia and urban Indonesia 1987 (Rp per capita per month) Quintiles of persons ranked by total household consumption per capita*

	Quintile 1	Quintile 2	Quintile 3	Quintile 4	Quintile 5	Average
All Indonesia						
Total per capita expenditure on health care of which:	85.48	116.34	148.80	232.72	378.48	192.37
Spent by household directly	21.84	39.08	49.28	89.72	224.52	84.89
Subsidy from government	63.64	77.26	99.52	143.00	153.96	107.48
Mean total consumption per capita	(9314.00)	(13,316.50)	(17,330.50)	(23,612.00)	(46,877.00)	(22,090.00)
Urban Indonesia						
Total per capita expenditure on health care of which:	146.63	245.96	266.94	236.56	533.38	296.33
Spent by household directly	44.26	86.76	113.54	153.61	373.69	154.38
Subsidy from government	102.37	159.20	153.39	82.95	159.69	141.95
Mean total consumption per capita	(3763.65.00)	(20,344.00)	(26,998.50)	(36,452.50)	(68,761.00)	(33,199.00)

Source: van de Walle, D. The distribution of the benefits from social services in Indonesia 1978–1987, *World Bank Policy Research Working Papers WPS 871,* The World Bank, Washington
Rp = Rupees

Table 6.3 *Treatment of illness – urban Indonesia 1987 (%)*
Quintiles of persons ranked by total household consumption per capita

Quintiles	1 (poorest)	2	3	4	5 (richest)
Urban Indonesia					
Last week's illness treated by:					
Private doctor	9.1	20.3	20.5	32.1	41.7
Hospital	6.4	10.5	11.5	11.0	15.7
Primary health centre	27.3	29.0	31.5	23.0	13.7
Polyclinic	3.2	1.0	3.3	3.1	2.3
Paramedic	13.7	10.7	2.4	5.4	3.3
Traditional healer	2.6	1.5	0.9	2.0	1.4
Self or family	31.7	23.3	24.5	19.9	20.6
No medication	5.9	3.7	3.9	3.6	1.3
Per cent of above receiving inpatient treatment	1.4	3.1	2.7	3.8	7.2
Inpatient at/with					
Primary health centre	19.6	4.2	14.1	17.5	7.1
Hospital	72.7	95.7	84.0	71.2	88.7
Paramedic	0.0	0.2	1.7	2.9	3.2
Traditional healer	7.7	0.0	0.2	8.5	1.1

Source: van de Walle, D (1992) The distribution of the benefits from social services in Indonesia 1978–1987, *World Bank Policy Research Working Papers* WPS 871, The World Bank, Washington DC.

income groups (Table 6.2) and that urban hospital facilities are likely to be used relatively more by wealthier people. Table 6.3 shows that over 15 per cent of the wealthiest 20 per cent of urban residents had their last illness treated in hospital compared with 6 per cent of the poorest 20 per cent. This is unlikely to be explained by severity of illness. Overall, in 1987 government subsidies for health care disproportionately benefited residents of urban areas. Forty one per cent of total subsidy was used in urban areas where only 27 per cent of the population reside (Table 6.4). However, some disproportion is not necessarily inequitable if it reflects functioning referral services.

This trend seems to have become more pronounced since 1978. However, some care has to be exercised in interpreting the numbers, as the proportion of the population located in urban areas is likely to have increased between the two dates.

Within urban areas of Indonesia, the distribution of health sector subsidies in urban areas appears to have become more equitable since 1978 (Table 6.4). More expenditure is now targeted at the poorest 40 per cent and less on the upper 30 per cent. Nonetheless this top group still commands 14 per cent of government health subsidy (down from 16 per cent). The middle 30 per cent band of urban households has also benefited (increasing its share from 5 per cent to 12 per cent).

Central government may further bias expenditure towards urban areas. In India, Rao et al (quoted in Griffin 1992) compared urban and rural expenditure on health and family welfare in 1983 (Table 6.5). The degree of bias varied considerably by state suggesting the potential for considerable discretion. For comparison, the urban bias which can be estimated from the data for Indonesia which was discussed above is 1.5.

Data from the Philippines suggest that the use of public health services may be more inequitable for urban than for rural facilities (Table 6.6). Some 30 per cent of the users of urban facilities were from the richest class compared with 20 per cent of the users of rural facilities.

Recent trends in the role of government finance have reflected the swiftly deteriorating economic, political and social climate that most developing countries have faced in the last few years. Many national economies and city administrations have suffered economic contraction and have had to cut annual spending plans.

A number of countries facing critical situations have undergone stabilization and structural adjustment programmes associated with the International Monetary Fund and the World Bank. These bring fundamental changes in the way the economy operates at both national and local level. Common features are devaluation of currencies, reduced government spending and reallocation of resources, contraction of public sector employment, changes in the prices of goods and services and measures to improve public sector efficiency.

The combination of economic recession and some aspects of these policies have resulted in falling standards of public services in many instances. Some symptoms may be lack of capital investment, deteriorating buildings and equipment, shortages of pharmaceutical and other supplies and a poor logistics system to deliver, supervise and support essential services like monitoring water quality. Phased maintenance and repairs to water and sewerage systems have been neglected. Many fully trained central and local government staff have moved to the private sector; less qualified staff have faced redundancy (Zulu and Nsouli 1985, Nicholas 1988, Thomas et al 1991).

The adjustment process has affected poverty and inequality in the city. Fragmentary evidence from Indonesia suggests that the urban sector has been more adversely affected than the rural sector (Ahmed 1991). In Mexico the deteriorating circumstances of the urban poor have been deliberately cushioned by government. As global subsidies were reduced, targeted subsidies were introduced for the poorest groups in the cities (Nash 1991).

State and city authorities

The expenditure responsibility of cities varies widely across countries and accurate data on the finances of individual local authorities are not collected by any central agency for purposes of international comparison (Bahl and Linn 1992). Bahl and Nath (1986) have attempted to estimate the expenditure share of sub-national governments (states and cities). On average, across countries, they estimated this as 15 per cent. In larger

Table 6.4 *Percentage shares of Indonesian government health subsidies by household expenditure groups, urban and rural areas 1987 (1978)*

Household expenditure group		Indonesia Urban	Rural	Total
Lower 40%	1987	15	16	31
	1978	(1)	(18)	(19)
Middle 30%	1987	12	17	29
	1978	(5)	(31)	(36)
Upper 30%	1987	14	25	39
	1978	(16)	(29)	(45)
Total	1987	41	58	100
	1978	(23)	(77)	(100)
Percentage share of population	1987	27	73	100
	1978	(19)	(81)	(100)

Source: van de Walle, D (1992). The distribution of the benefits from social services in Indonesia, 1978–1987, *World Bank Policy Research Working Papers* WPS 871, The World Bank, Washington DC.

metropolitan areas this figure rises to 30–50 per cent. Around this average there is substantial variation but it emphasises the important role city governments play in the provision of urban services and in the economic development of cities.

National governments finance part of a city's expenditure usually through a number of hybrid financing arrangements such as grants and revenue sharing. Central government usually makes intergovernmental transfers to reduce inequalities between regions and cities. Central government may also seek to compensate cities which incur high costs such as those which have to deal with exceptional levels of overcrowding or particular social problems. The level of central government transfers to cities to recurrent expenditure in eight countries is shown in Table 6.7.

The distinction between external funds and locally raised revenues is an important one because it is an indicator of the self-sufficiency of urban

Table 6.5 *Distribution of health and family welfare expenditure between urban and rural areas in India 1983 (%)*

	Urban	Rural	Common	Urban bias[a]
State governments	41.1	18.6	40.3	2.6
Central government	55.4	0.9	43.7	–
All India	44.0	15.1	40.9	2.3

Note:
a) % total budget allocated to urban areas/% total population resident in urban areas
Source: Adapted from: Rao, Kahn and Prasad (1987) Health sector expenditure differentials in India Ministry of Health and Family Welfare, Baroda quoted in Griffin C (1992) Healthcare in Asia: a comparative study of costs and financing, The World Bank, Washington DC

Table 6.6 *The Philippines: use of public health facilities by income class*

| | use of public facility[a] | |
Income class	Rural	Hospital health unit
Lower	38%	31%
Middle	34%	35%
Upper	20%	30%
Other (unclassified)	8%	4%

Note:
a) Percentage of users from the different income classes
Source: Solon et al 1991 Health sector financing in the Philippines. Research Triangle Institute and University of the Philippines School of Economics, quoted in WHO (1993) Evaluation of recent changes in the financing of health services, WHO, Geneva, Switzerland

administrations. There is an assumption that the city has more discretion in managing its own revenue. The share of locally raised revenues in financing city expenditure has varied from 100 per cent in Karachi to 27 per cent in Kinshasa in recent years. The locally financed share has declined significantly in the 1980s (Bahl and Linn 1992). Cities have relied on traditional instruments of charging and taxation and have been slow and ineffective in chasing defaulters. In five out of eight countries where municipal revenue was analyzed by the World Bank, locally raised revenue was less than 50 per cent of the total (Table 6.7).

Table 6.7 *Sources of recurrent municipal revenue – selected countries (%)[b]*

	Central transfers	Local taxes[a]	Local fees and charges
India	65	10	25
Indonesia	8	9	84
Kenya	39	55	6
Tunisia	32	13	54
Turkey	9	29	62
Brazil	23	9	68
Colombia	44	14	42
Mexico	12	25	64

Notes:
a) Includes property taxes collected by central government and returned to municipal governments on the basis of origin
b) Excludes receipts from borrowing and capital grants
Source: World Bank (1991) Urban policy and economic development: an agenda for the 1990s, The World Bank, Washington DC

The sources of city revenues differ. Local taxes usually have a smaller impact on redistribution of wealth than central taxes. The most important local tax is the property tax (Table 6.8). There are usually only crude equations between the value of residential property and the incomes of owners and occupiers. The relation between the value of commercial property in a city and the relative profitability of business is even more tenuous. Nonetheless, most cities retain property taxes and many are currently revitalizing them (revaluation, betterment taxes, property transfer taxes) to try to ensure a fairly reliable source of revenue (Davey and Devas 1992).

Expenditure taxes are also common and less redistributive than income taxes, which are also used, since the ratio of expenditure to income falls as income rises. Other forms of local taxation include taxes on goods entering a city for consumption or processing, transaction taxes, business occupational taxes and consumption taxes.

In addition, city authorities may charge for services. Health services usually incur only small charges with some types of health services such as immunization and family planning often exempted. Water, sewerage, and other services are generally considered more suitable for charging, and are frequently provided on a full cost recovery basis. Table 6.8 shows that for the seven cities for which data are available, refuse collection incurs a deficit and therefore needs subsidy from public funds. Some charges such as those for licences to sell food or water may have a primary purpose of regulating and recording the activity rather than cost recovery.

The most sophisticated current analyses of demand for health, water and sanitation and municipal services provided on a fee for service basis take account of both monetary costs and the cost of obtaining care or a service in terms of a user's time. The city dweller is better placed as there are usually a range of facilities within reach. However, the poorest city dwellers may lack access to even the most basic services, and time costs (for fetching water) as well as increased charges (for medical care) may mean that they decide to use services less or not at all. Data from Indonesia show a strong relationship between a low level of income and the likelihood of being treated only within the family and of receiving no medication when becoming ill (Table 6.3).

Charges may contribute to regressivity of service provision. A World Bank case study of metropolitan Manila revealed a wide variation in per capita expenditures amongst the 17 constituent local government units (Bahl et al 1976). The wealthiest areas often receive more. For example, Makati, the wealthiest of the municipalities, contained about 2 per cent of the total municipal population in 1975 but produced about 41 per cent of municipal revenues (including non-charge revenue). It was a well serviced area. There are considerable disparities in service levels within the urban area – low income neighbourhoods with less ability to pay for services do not have the same access to services as do high income neighbourhoods. It should be noted that this situation at least implies greater progressivity of financing than where similar access inequities exist in a tax financed system.

A final source of finance at subnational level is the raising of loans and issuing of bonds. This is usually for financing capital development.

City administrations also vary widely with respect to the use of revenues raised. For example, expenditure directly on health services themselves varies from 0.8 per cent in Seoul to 24.4 per cent in Karachi (Table 6.9). Within health related expenditure, emphasis also differs. The most common functions of city administrations appear to be running public health facilities below hospital level, street cleaning and rubbish collection, and regulation of markets and abattoirs. In certain cases city administrations have full or partial responsibility for the construction and

Table 6.8 *Financing of solid waste collection in selected cities*

City (year)	Refuse charges		Financial status
	Residential	*Industrial/commercial*	
Bogotá, Colombia (1973)	Property tax surcharge	Tax on business value, and volume charge above minimum level	Deficit
Cartagena, Colombia (1973)	Property tax surcharge (non-earmarked)	Property tax surcharge (non-earmarked)	Deficit (tax less than expenditure for refuse collection)
Ahmadabad, India (1972)	Conservancy tax (non-earmarked property tax surcharge)	Conservancy tax	Deficit (tax less than expenditure for refuse collection)
Bombay, India (1974)	Conservancy tax (non-earmarked property tax surcharge)	Conservancy tax	Deficit (tax less than expenditure for refuse collection)
Jakarta, Indonesia (1973)	None	Private collection and disposal, except where special contract with public agency	–
Kingston Jamaica (1974)	None	None	
Seoul, Rep. of Korea (1973)	Flat monthly charge varying with household space, monthly income and property value	Flat volume charge	Deficit
Singapore (1974)	Flat monthly charge, except in public housing, where no charge	Commercial – flat monthly charge plus volume surcharge for collection above minimum volume; industrial – private collection, with free disposal at public sites	Deficit
Tunis, Tunisia (1974)	Sanitation tax (non-earmarked surcharge on rental tax)	Sanitation tax (non-earmarked surcharge on rental tax)	Deficit (tax less than expenditure for refuse collection)

Source: Bahl, R W O and Linn, J F (1992) Urban finance in developing countries. The World Bank, Washington DC Oxford University Press

maintenance of a potable water supply, sewerage and drainage. Larger cities usually have a greater range of responsibilities than smaller cities (Bahl and Linn 1992). Quite frequently responsibilities for certain services are devolved to autonomous local public agencies. It is not at all unusual for an agency to account for more than one-third of total local government expenditure. The responsibility for supplying water, in particular, is frequently dealt with this way (Table 6.10).

PRIVATE SOURCES OF FINANCE

The previous section emphasized the extent of information shortage concerning public sources of finance. However, this is insignificant when compared with the lack of information about private sources. In the private sector, information has to be collated from a number of sources most of which are not routine and many of which are likely to be systematically biased.

A number of cities have included in their policies a degree of commitment to expand the private sector and to involve more private capital. Some current examples of new ways of working are a willingness to liberalize the conditions under which staff may practise privately, sometimes using public facilities to do so; contracting out of services such as refuse collection in the city, or laundry or catering services in the hospital; purchase of pieces of diagnostic equipment in the private health sector being shared with the public sector on a fee for service basis. In other cities the private sector is growing without any change in policy or government incentives because people increasingly appear to be prepared to pay for quality and privacy, particularly those who are better off. The increased use of charges in the public sector which has already been discussed may be a further factor which has led to a shift to the private sector.

Private spending in Indonesia, for example, accounts for over half of all expenditures on health. People in urban areas spend more on health care than those in the rural areas. The richest 20 per cent of the urban population spend 3.65 times as much on health care as the poorest 20 per cent (Table 6.2).

Some data from Indonesia showing utilization of the services of private doctors in urban areas was presented in Table 6.3. The percentage of reported illnesses treated by private doctors ranges from 9 per cent for the poorest 20 per cent of the population to 42 per cent for the richest 20 per cent. The poorest tend to seek care at public primary health care centres: of the poorest 20 per cent some 27 per cent seek care there compared with 14 per cent of the richest 20 per cent.

The scope and objectives of privatization policies have varied considerably. Most cities have witnessed some degree of privatization. In health care, in areas where there was limited capacity to provide services such as mental health care, terminal care and care of the elderly, and both central and city administrations were aware of the lacunae in services, the private sector has been encouraged to play a more active role. Non–governmental and charitable organizations have been encouraged to shoulder responsibilities for some of these activities.

Table 6.9 *Percentage distribution of total expenditure of local authorities by function in selected cities of nine developing countries (%)*

Function	Columbia Cali (1974)	India Ahmadabad (1981)	Jamaica Kingston (1972)	Korea Seoul (1983)	Zambia Lusaka (1972)	Brazil São Paulo (1984)	Kenya Nairobi (1981)	Pakistan Karachi (1982)	Philippines Manila (1985)
Public utility of which:	**50.2**	**17.6**	**3.8**	**9.2**	**26.9**	**26.1**	–	**21.6**	–
Water supply	12.3	12.0	3.8	8.1	21.1	–	31.8	11.6	–
Sewerage/drainage	–	5.6	–	1.0	5.8	–	–	–	–
Social services of which:	**3.5**	**32.0**	**17.0**	**40.6**	**15.4**	**51.4**	**41.0**	**30.8**	**51.4**
Health	1.8	10.6	5.0	0.8	3.3	8.2	18.9	24.4	7.2
Transportation	**6.0**	**8.2**	**23.5**	**16.3**	**5.3**	**18.5**	**6.8**	**30.7**	**0.1**
General urban services of which:	**3.9**	**9.5**	**39.4**	**7.6**	**20.5**	**0.4**	–	**7.4**	**12.4**
Refuse collection	2.4	5.4	23.3	–	2.1	–	–	–	–
Markets and abattoirs	1.5	0.1	4.4	–	0.3	–	–	–	–
Other expenditure	36.5	32.6	16.4	26.3	31.9	29.8	20.3	9.4	36.0
Per capita expenditure (dollars)	51.4	n.a.	20.7	n.a.	63.1	56.0	58.3	n.a.	5.8

Note:
n.a. not available
Source: Bahl, R W and Linn, J F (1992) Urban public finance in developing countries, The World Bank, Washington DC, Oxford University Press

Table 6.10 Percentage contribution of autonomous local agencies to consolidated local government spending in selected cities

City, Year	Number of agencies	Percentage of total expenditure	Percentage of capital expenditure	Autonomous agency functions
Botswana				
Francistown, 1972	2	39.9	n.a.	Water, electricity
Colombia				
Bogotá, 1972	12	79.3	98.5	Public utilities, housing, roads, public transportation, refuse collection
Cali, 1974	4	80.0	90.9	Public utilities, housing, roads, refuse collection
Cartagena, 1972	4	84.1	84.4	Public utilities, roads, refuse collection
India				
Ahmadabad, 1971	3	58.7	32.7	Education, public transportation, milk scheme
Bombay, 1972	1	30.2	19.7	Electricity, public transportation
Bombay, 1982	1	39.2	19.4	–
Indonesia				
Jakarta, 1972	5	23.2	15.9	Water, public transportation, land development, education, abattoir
Jakarta, 1982	4	11.0	–	–
Jamaica				
Kingston, 1972	1[a]	43.4	73.4	Water

Korea, Republic of				
Daegu, 1975	n.a.	42.2	–	Water, land readjustment, housing
Daegu, 1983		35.4		
Daejeon, 1975	n.a.	38.4	–	Water, land readjustment, housing
Daejeon, 1983		45.4		
Gwangju, 1975	n.a.	21.6	–	Water, land readjustment, housing
Gwangju, 1983		65.6		
Jeonju, 1975	n.a.	36.0	–	Water, land readjustment, housing
Jeonju, 1983		40.5		
Seoul, 1971	1	23.1	10.3	Education
Seoul, 1983	1	25.5	39.1	–
Nicaragua				
Managua, 1974	1	28.7[b]	–	Water
Managua, 1979	1	25.1	–	–

Notes: – not applicable   n.a. not available   a) Based on revenues

Source: Bahl R W and Linn J F (1992) Urban public finance in developing countries, World Bank, Washington DC, Oxford University Press

There is a question mark over the potential of private sector financing to raise further revenues for health, water and sanitation or municipal services. Economic recession affecting many cities has meant that people have less money available to pay fees. Fewer savings are available for private sector initiatives such as building a clinic or bidding to take control of a refuse collection service with its concomitant investment in expensive vehicles and site provision. However, privatization is likely to have greater potential in urban than in rural areas. City dwellers have greater opportunities for employment in the formal sector and are likely to be paid in cash. They are more used to a monetized economy and are more likely to be able to afford to pay than those who live in rural areas. Demand has been observed to recover in urban areas in Ghana after charges have been imposed (Waddington and Enyimayew 1989).

Little evidence is available as yet as to whether a greater role for the private sector increases efficiency. There is some evidence to suggest that many private providers of basic services eg a medical practitioner or a hospital laundry service may provide services more cheaply than the public sector. However, the quality and type of services offered may not always be the same. Vendors who supply water to cities may offer inferior quality, and commonly make higher charges than public providers (Table 6.11). Other data confirm this finding. Ratios of private to public water costs are, in Abidjan 5:1; for selected cities in Indonesia, between 2:1 and 10:1 (World Bank data); in Karachi 10:1 (USAID data); and in Lima between 16:1 and 25:1 (quoted in Bahl and Linn 1992). In the Klong Toey slum in Bangkok, the cost of private water per month is equivalent to four days' wages (World Bank 1991). Contractual arrangements may promote or worsen efficiency depending on a number of factors such as the size of a city and the level of development of its infrastructure (McPake 1994). Competition may lead to greater concern with internal efficiency. However, there are costs attached to establishing proper mechanisms for the private sector to tender to operate services, and for the quality of services offered to be monitored and assessed. There is a need for further procedures for termination of services where those rendered have been unsatisfactory, and also re-tendering systems put in place.

While quality of services is difficult to measure, it might be assumed that where privatization introduces consumer choice, some aspects of quality are likely to improve. Nevertheless, there are clear exceptions to this, particularly in the pharmaceutical sector where examples of poor quality services from private enterprises are well documented (White 1991, Yesudian 1994).

Another cause for concern is that as the private sector grows in size and importance and the better off seek to use more private services and minimize their use of public services, much of the well argued and constructive criticism of public services that acts as a spur to change and improvement will be lost. Two tier systems can lead to inferior services being permanently on offer to poor people.

The equity effects of both user fees, and promotion of the private sector in taking on an enhanced role in providing services, wholly, or in part, depend on national or city commitment to redirecting extra revenue gained to improve services overall or to provide services to the poorest

Table 6.11 *Costs of public and private water supply in selected developing countries ($ per m³)*

Country or city	In-house connection (public utility)	Water carrier (private vendor)
Burkina Faso	0.30	1.0–1.5
Ghana	0.10	1.3–2.5
Nairobi, Kenya	0.20	1.4–2.1
Senegal	Free	1.6–2.4
Kampala, Uganda	0.33	1.3–3.0

Source: Data from Linn and Vlieger quoted in Bahl and Linn (1992) Urban public finance in developing countries, The World Bank, Washington DC, Oxford University Press

groups. These new services in the poorest parts of the city may have to be heavily subsidized. Attention must be given to the acceptability of private payments to politicians and users. Charges have been more unattractive historically to national rather than local politicians. Cities have a long history of collecting revenues, fees and taxes from a local population and have a greater degree of manoeuvrability. The acceptance of the notion of charging by the inhabitants of a city appears to be linked to greater availability of cash, their closeness to the services, and their acute perception of the quality of services they are receiving.

INSURANCE

Insurance is usually at least a 'bipartite' if not 'tripartite' source of finance in that it normally involves contributions from employers and employees and often also from government. Thus it is neither a purely public nor purely private source.

A proportion of a city's population will have health care costs covered by health insurance schemes. In much of Africa and Asia the scope for compulsory health insurance was long thought to be severely limited because of the smaller percentage of the city population that worked in the formal as compared with the informal sector. However, a review in 1982 showed that more than half of all low and middle income developing counties have some form of medical insurance as part of a social security system (Zschock 1982). Most schemes are concentrated in the industrial sector and are to be found in cities (Mills 1983).

An examination of the number of people entitled to health benefits in Phit Sanulok Municipality, Thailand showed that 48.3 per cent of the population was not covered by any scheme (Table 6.12). The high percentage of civil servants covered by schemes reflected the large bureaucracy in the town and partly also the sampling technique. The most disadvantaged groups without cover tended to be those in the lowest occupational and income groups and to come from farming, semi-skilled jobs and trading and service activities (Pannarunothai 1992).

Many national governments have reconsidered their positions and are now re-examining the viability of plans to establish compulsory health insurance schemes because of their own limited resources.

Health insurance premiums are earmarked for health expenditure and are unlikely to be diverted to other purposes. The level of resources raised depends on whether the scheme covering a city's population is part of a national scheme or whether it is partial, specific to certain types of employees. Another consideration is whether the scheme is run on a for profit or non profit basis. The larger the proportion of the population in the informal economy, the more difficult it is to raise contributions. During periods of recession, unemployment is likely to rise and real wages to decrease. This can affect the level of resources available to the insurance scheme.

Concern is often expressed that health insurance schemes may not work well from the point of view of allocative efficiency. Too many resources are often devoted to curative care, particularly private doctors and hospital care (Kutzin and Barnum 1992), and too much may be spent on a small proportion of the city's population. Research in Brazil indicated that in 1981 total expenditure on 12,000 high cost patients enrolled in INAMPS (the health insurance component of Brazil's payroll financial social security system) was greater than the amount spent to provide basic health services and disease control for 41 million people in the poor north and northeast regions of the country (McGreevey 1988). Administrative efficiency is also a cause for concern. Administrative costs may absorb a high percentage of insurance premiums. A further factor that can affect efficient working is the structure and functioning of liaison mechanisms with the Ministry of Health.

Criticism of the equity effects of health insurance schemes is frequently directed at the fact that it is urban wage-earners and their dependants who are usually covered. This better off group is covered by an extensive range of benefits of which the recipients may themselves fund only a third or less. Thus the central government or the employer subsidizes health care for the better off in the city.

DONOR ASSISTANCE

This final source of finance to be considered here, like insurance, contains both public and private elements. The greatest part is bilateral and multilateral aid. This type of expenditure is most commonly included within government accounts, often not separately identified. The private component is that of donations from charitable organizations. These are usually channelled through Non-governmental organizations (NGOs) which play a significant role particularly in health services in many countries. Donations usually provide part of the finances of NGOs, alongside government contributions and the revenues from direct payments (Dave-Sen and McPake 1993).

The OECD reported that an average of 5.3 per cent of total bilateral agency assistance in 1988 was for health and population activities; such activities accounted for 6.1 per cent of World Bank funding and 19.1 per cent of United Nations specialized agency funding (OECD 1989). The actual level of funding and its disposal over the years of a project is often difficult to ascertain as donor agencies usually set out their projects and

Table 6.12 *Phit Sanulok Municipality, Thailand – health benefits by household income group (% of population)*

Quintile group	Not covered	Civil servant	State enterprise	Veteran volunteer	Low income	Social security	Private employer	Private insurance
1	69.7	14.65	0.55	1.70	6.75	0.4	1.3	4.3
2	57.5	30.75	0.75	1.95	2.7	1.4	1.3	3.4
3	48.2	34.45	3.9	2.15	3.0	0.7	1.6	5.7
4	33.5	51.85	5.55	1.25	0.6	1.3	2.45	3.4
5	35.85	44.25	8.7	1.50	0.3	1.1	1.5	5.8
Unknown	69.2	16.7	5.1	0.6	0.0	0.0	0.0	8.3
Total	**48.3**	**35.8**	**4.3**	**1.7**	**2.3**	**0.9**	**1.6**	**4.7**

Sources: Pannarunothai, P (1992) *Equity in Health: The Need for and Use of Public and Private Health Services in Phitsanulok Municipality* Ministry of Public Health (Provincial Hospital Division), Bangkok, Thailand

programmes on a country basis without breaking down activities to the level of individual cities.

External finance may promote allocative efficiency by devoting resources to priority action such as water supply, sanitation or primary health services and increasing coverage of the population. However, the practice of funding capital or development expenditure only has aggravated allocative inefficiency in some cases by encouraging larger schemes than might have been necessary or sustainable within a city. In addition, this strategy has sometimes led to imbalance in financing with capital structures insufficiently maintained and under-utilized. Donors have increased their willingness to fund recurrent costs for these reasons in recent years.

The technical and administrative efficiency of externally financed projects may often be higher than those run by national or city governments because of the input of highly qualified expatriate staff. The greater problem often arises in sustaining this level of operation after the donor withdraws.

Targeting the urban poor is often a primary concern of donor-led projects. Designing these actions, costing them, and assessing their effectiveness in improving health status has been seriously hampered by the lack of socio-economic data in most cities, particularly data on income distribution and consumption patterns. City specific data bases are needed, given the wide diversity of situations and the different foci in the design of antipoverty programmes.

The lack of information regarding donor activities and donor expenditure may make coordination by city authorities virtually impossible. City planners are left with no overall picture of the purpose, location or amount of funds flowing into a city. More attention needs to be given to ensure that projects are known and are acceptable both to the donor and to the city. The need for urban strategic planning is self-evident.

CONCLUSIONS

From the information which has been compiled in this chapter, it is possible to reach a number of tentative conclusions regarding some of the major issues affecting urban health related services. There are a large number of sources of finance for services in urban areas, a greater diversity than found elsewhere. This causes some planning difficulties but may also increase the stability of funding levels overall. Even within the public sector, there are central and local sources and various Ministries and local authority departments involved. All these sources appear to be characterized by a substantial degree of inequity where data are available. The private sector appears to be increasing in scope and scale in most countries but it is not clear that private sector financing is either more efficient or more equitable. A number of countries are re-examining the feasibility of insurance arrangements. These need to be planned carefully to avoid problems of allocative efficiency and government subsidy of relatively prosperous groups. The principal problems associated with donor assistance appear to be its *ad hoc* nature, sustainability and coordination.

However, a critical problem, apparent from the preceding sections, is the gap in information at present. The main gaps are discussed below. The annex to this chapter proposes an outline protocol which city authorities may consider using in order to provide the missing information needed for effective planning and management. The aim should be to identify broad orders of magnitude rather than to account for all expenditures precisely. Low cost and swift studies are to be preferred to meticulous and protracted studies that can rapidly become out of date. While such a study will consume resources, this chapter has argued that the information provided is essential for effective planning and management of urban health related services. If its results are used judiciously, it should prove a productive investment.

It is difficult to establish the amount spent by government and other agencies and to link expenditure with health status. There is almost no information on expenditure targeted at poor people and the health outcome for the high risk groups. While most donors aim to promote PHC and services for poorer groups, information on the contribution of each type of funder, the types of services provided and the geographical and socio-economic distribution of users is essential if these problems are to be overcome.

Little information was available on the total expenditure made by households in a city on health, water and sanitation and environmental services. The information may be collected on a national basis for Family Expenditure Surveys in some countries. It could then be disaggregated to give information regarding individual cities. The extent to which increased use of direct charges and the private sector alters the level and distribution of expenditures and service use is therefore unknown in the urban context. Some evidence of inaccessibility for poor groups in the context of a range of services and prices was presented from the Philippines. If such problems are to be avoided, planners need this information.

Private payments for services, privatization of services and supplies, and entrepreneurial development of new services all signal a far greater role for the private sector. However, little is known about the extent of private sector activities, the types or quality of services involved or the users of those services. Where city authorities are directly encouraging growth of private sector activities, this information will be needed for effective monitoring and regulation.

The problem of providing insurance cover for people in poorly paid jobs in the formal sector and for people in the informal sector remains unsolved. While more information is usually available about levels of coverage of insurance companies and their patterns of expenditure, little may be known about the utilization patterns of those covered and the implications of extending insurance arrangements to the uncovered. The appropriateness of public contributions to insurance schemes can only be judged in this context.

Many cities obtain substantial donor funding across different sectors. The money may be spent within the city but administratively may be dealt with by agencies outside, such as central government ministries or Non-governmental organizations. One of the major problems identified with donor funding in urban areas is the difficulty of coordinating and integrating activities with those of others. Information on volume of funds, types of services provided and geographical and socio-economic distribution of users is needed before coordination can even begin. However, differing project accounting classifications and methods of dispersal of funds mean that special analysis has to be undertaken to work out the amount of funds intended for a city and the many heads under which the expenditure takes place.

ANNEX:
OUTLINE PROTOCOL TO ASSESS THE FINANCING
SITUATION OF HEALTH SERVICES IN A CITY

Tables A, B and C identify the information which the chapter has suggested should be collected.

When considering the way to collect financial data which can provide a comprehensive picture of expenditure, there are a number of important points to remember, not least that no central accounting system in the city is keeping track of the total amounts being spent. It is important:

- To ensure that all the data collected relates to the same financial year.
- To use actual expenditure, and not budgeted figures. Audited figures would be even preferable but there may be delays before these are produced.
- To make certain that all major categories of expenditure are included. Expenditure in the private sector may prove elusive and difficult.
- To check that there is no double counting.
- To check that book transfers are not recorded as actual expenditures.
- To collect capital as well as recurrent expenditure, wherever possible. Failure to account for public capital can lead to serious underestimation of the total public resources used to provide services. If possible several years' previous capital expenditure should be calculated and averaged, as capital expenditure tends to be 'lumpy'. Knowledge of capital expenditure is important to policy decisions.

The relative usefulness of using rough as opposed to detailed estimates can be argued. The main purpose in attempting the exercise is to equip policy makers and management with relevant financial information so that they can plan and take decisions which will promote the overall well-being of the city and its inhabitants. The purpose, therefore, has to be balanced against the cost. It is for the individual city to decide how much it is prepared to spend. To keep costs low, and to establish a system of working that would allow the data to be drawn together annually, researchers should try to use existing sources of information and accounting systems, even where these present substantial difficulties. The alternative – to initiate basic research – or to attempt to revise central government or municipal accounting systems may not be justified on a benefit-cost basis.

Ministry of Health

The Ministry will usually have responsibility for running large tertiary or secondary hospitals in the city. The layout of the budget will need to be checked to establish if expenditure is recorded on a facility basis. If so, it will make expenditure fairly easy to retrieve. Other Ministries may have responsibilities in relation to the hospitals, eg Ministry of Works for maintenance, Ministry of Transport for vehicles.

Other central Ministries (Ministry of Water, Ministry of Local Government etc)

In all cities health and health related expenditures will be made by Ministries other than the Ministry of Health. The Ministry of Water may have responsibility for construction of dams and piping water to city boundaries. The Ministry of Local Government may have responsibility for all training of city personnel above a certain cadre of staff.

Other Ministries may be spending directly on health in a city, eg the Ministry of Defence might have a barracks within the city and be spending on health services for the troops stationed there; the Ministry of Education may be spending on health education.

Appropriate enquiries need to be made to try to bring all the financial data relating to expenditure together.

State/city administrations

In countries with a federal structure of government, state administrations may have responsibility for running general hospitals in cities and for training all staff below the level of doctor. The city administrations may have responsibility for running municipal health centres and clinics only.

City administrations may have responsibility for transmission and distribution of water, and for sewerage systems. They normally run all rubbish collection and disposal systems and are responsible for enforcing many public health measures, such as pollution and effluent control, hygiene in shops and markets etc.

Health insurance

Most cities in developing countries have a proportion of people in stable jobs who are protected against most of the costs of medical care. These schemes may include government employees and those employed in parastatals, eg railway companies. Other health insurance schemes may provide private cover on an annual basis to individuals. The expenditures on private practitioners, private hospitals, pharmacies and private beds in public facilities is often large and is quite separate from the expenditure of the Ministry of Health. Cash benefits paid to sick persons should be excluded.

Private expenditures

This is the most difficult area of expenditure on which to acquire financial data, particularly in relation to expenditures on health care and pharmaceuticals. Data can be acquired in two ways – from the urban household itself or from the suppliers of services.

For the first method, data may be available from a National Household Income and Expenditure Survey. The data could then be extrapolated to the city situation. Specific surveys or samples might have been carried out by a city university undertaking research. Specific research for the city study is best avoided because of the time and cost involved.

A different approach is to ask the principal providers of services such as physicians, dentists, pharmacies (health), private suppliers of water or sewage removal services (water and sanitation) or private collectors of rubbish (environmental services) to give information on their earnings or takings. Professional associations are often willing to provide assistance with supplying names and addresses of members. Confidentiality and anonymity normally have to be guaranteed for financial information to be disclosed. Approaches to government tax departments are normally unsuccessful; they are reluctant to disclose earnings or discuss tax matters of individuals.

Special problems attach to estimating earnings of traditional practitioners, and herbalists. It is useful if either central government or the city administration has required registration of these practitioners. Enquiries can then be made as to level of charges and estimates made of the number of patients or customers.

Voluntary labour should be included under this heading. Volunteers often help out at city hospitals with nursing and other tasks.

Employers

Industrial and agro-processing plants often provide health services directly to their employees. The services are typically financed by the business concern and may cover the workers' families as well as the employees themselves.

Non-governmental organizations/charities/community groups

Donations often support health, water and sanitation and other public health activities. The largest sources of funds are very often foreign religious oganizations operating small hospitals or health services. Foreign developmental agencies often operate special projects and programmes to help the poorest groups in a city, sometimes linked with a national branch of the same agency.

In collecting financial data, separate account must be taken of funds from abroad and national funds (to avoid double counting). Payments by patients or users of services may also be an important source of income for NGOs and charities.

Donors

External development aid often has a significant part to play in a city's health promoting activities. Aid may be given on a multilateral basis (WHO, UNICEF, World Bank etc) or on a bilateral basis. Donors have been enthusiastic about supporting basic health services such as immunization and the development of water and sanitation systems. The financial information may be kept by the donors themselves or in the office of UNDP. Estimates may have to be made in relation to expenditure within a city on an immunization or an AIDS programme as the data are often kept centrally by a vertically organized programme.

Table A *Recurrent expenditure on health, water and sanitation and environmental services in 1994*

	National	State (province)	Local government	Private for profit	Mission/ voluntary/ donor
HEALTH SERVICES					
Primary health services					
Secondary health services					
Tertiary health services					
WATER AND SANITATION					
Water supply					
Sanitation					
ENVIRONMENTAL SERVICES					
Waste disposal etc					

Table B *Public capital expenditure and capital expenditure intentions relating to health, water and sanitation and environmental projects*

	1994 Forecast	1994 Actual	1995 Forecast	1996 Forecast	1997 Forecast
Total – million					
Inflation: % increase in actual/assumed prices compared with the previous year					
Amounts in total in: Health					
Water					
Sanitation					
Environment					

Table C *Recurrent expenditure on health, water and sanitation and environmental services: geographic and socio-economic distribution*

Distribution of expenditure	National	State (province)	Local govern- ment	Private for profit	Mission/ voluntary/ donor
GEOGRAPHIC					
Zone A					
Zone B					
.					
.					
.					
Zone X					
SOCIO-ECONOMIC GROUP					
Anticipated/ targeted users					
Socio-economic group 1					
Socio-economic group 2					
.					
.					
.					
Socio-economic group X					

REFERENCES

Ahmed, S (1991) Indonesia: stabilization and structural change, in Thomas, V et al (eds) *Restructuring Economies in Distress: Policy Reform and the World Bank*, Washington DC, The World Bank

Bahl, R Brigg, P Smith, R (1976) Urban public finances in developing countries: a case study of Metropolitan Manila *Urban and Regional Report* 77–8 Washington DC, The World Bank

Bahl, R, Linn, J (1992) *Urban Public Finance in Developing Countries* Oxford University Press, Washington DC, The World Bank

Bahl R W, Nath S (1986) Public expenditure decentralization in developing countries. *Government & Policy* 4: 405–418

Bennett, S (1991) The mystique of markets: public and private healthcare in developing countries. PHP Departmental Publication: 4. London, London School of Hygiene and Tropical Medicine

Davey, K Devas N (1992) Urban government finance. Working Paper: 4, The institutional framework of urban management Development Administration Group (DAG), Institute of Local Government Studies, University of Birmingham, UK.

Dave-Sen, P McPake, B (1993) Planning and management of community financing: a review of NGO approaches in the health sector *Voluntas*, 4, 3: 326–371

De Ferranti, D (1985) Paying for health services in developing countries *World Bank Staff Working Papers* 721, The World Bank, Washington DC

Griffin, C C (1992) *Healthcare in Asia: A Comparative Study of Costs and Financing* The World Bank, Washington DC

Kutzin, J Barnum, H (1992) How health insurance affects the delivery of healthcare in developing countries *Policy Research Working Paper* WPS 852. Washington DC, The World Bank

McGreevey, W P (1988) The high costs of healthcare in Brazil. *PAHO Bulletin* 22 (2):145–166.

McPake, B (1994) Contracting out of health services in developing countries. *Health Policy and Planning* 9 (1): 25–30

Mills, A (1983) Economic aspects of health insurance in Lee, K and Mills, A (eds), *The Economics of Health in Developing Countries* Oxford University Press Oxford, UK.

Nash, J (1991) Mexico: adjustment and stabilization. In Thomas, V et al *Restructuring Economies in Distress: Policy Reform and the World Bank* Washington, The World Bank.

Nicholas, P (1988) The World Bank's lending for adjustment: an interim report. *World Bank Discussion Papers* No 34 Washington DC, The World Bank

OECD (1989) *Development Co-operation in the 1990s* Paris, France: Organization for Economic Co-operation and Development

Pannarunothai, S (1992) *Equity in Health: The Need for and Use of Public and Private Services in Phitsanulok Municipality*. Bangkok, Thailand: Ministry of Public Health (Provincial Hospital Division)

Solon, O et al (1991) *Health Sector Financing in the Philippines* Manila, The Philippines: Research Triangle Institute and University of the Philippines School of Economics

Thomas, V et al (eds) (1991) *Restructuring Economies in Distress: Policy Reform and the World Bank* World Bank, Washington, DC. Oxford University Press, New York

Van de Walle, D (1992) The distribution of the benefits from social services in Indonesia *World Bank Policy Research Working Papers* WPS 871 Washington, DC The World Bank.

Waddington, C Enyimayew, K (1989) A price to pay: the impact of user charges in Ashanti Akim District, Ghana *International Journal of Health Planning and Management* 4: pp17–47

White, S (1991) Medicines and self-help: the privatization of healthcare in Eastern Uganda in Hanson, H and Twaddle, M (eds) *Changing Uganda* Eastern Africa Studies Series James Currey, London

World Bank (1991) *Urban Policy and Economic Development: an Agenda for the 1990s* The World Bank, Washington DC

World Health Organization (1991) *The Public/Private Mix in National Health Systems and the Role of Ministries of Health. Report of an InterRegional Meeting, Mexico, July 1991,* WHO/SHS/NHP/91.2 World Health Organization, Geneva

World Health Organization (1993) *Evaluation of Recent Changes in the Financing of Health Services*, World Health Organization, Geneva

Yesudian, C (1994) Behaviour of the private sector in the health market in Bombay *Health Policy and Planning* pp72–80

Zschock, D (1982) General review of problems of medical care delivery under social security in developing countries *Int Soc Sec Rev* XXXV (1/82), pp3–15.

Zulu, J Nsouli, S 1985) *Adjustment Programs in Africa: the Recent Experience* Occasional Paper no 34, International Monetary Fund, Washington DC

7

How the World Health Organization Supports Urban Health Development

*Greg Goldstein, Allessandro Rossi-Espagnet
and Iraj Tabibzadeh*

INTRODUCTION

Involvement in activities related to the health effects of urbanization and the development of urban health systems went through a long gestational period in WHO primarily related to the fact that, until recently, priority, if not exclusive attention, was given to the problems of rural populations. During the last decade, however, increasing attention has been given to urban health development which has now become one of the important priorities of WHO and involves practically all technical programmes. This chapter specifically refers to the work of the Organization related to the strengthening of urban health services and the improvement of the urban environment.

STRENGTHENING OF URBAN HEALTH SERVICES

In 1963, an Expert Committee on Urban Health Services (WHO 1963) attempted to capture the universal dimension and the drama of urbanization that was unfolding in most cities of the developing world. It pointed out that 'the consequences of explosive growth of cities threaten to become one of the major problems of our age' and it emphasized that 'by tradition, the planning of cities has been an architectural function, but that it needs to be regarded more and more as a cooperative effort which takes into account not only the physical and economic aspects but also the social and environmental factors'.

A similar attempt was subsequently made at a meeting on the 'Health Effects of Urbanization' convened a few years later (WHO 1970). Although the resulting report could be considered as a good framework for a research programme in that area (which, in fact, is what it had been intended to be) and although some valuable points were made (see, for example, the discussion on intra-urban differentiation), it lacked the sense of urgency that the topic, should already have deserved at that time. It is not, therefore, surprising that a programme of activities formulated at about the same time by the same WHO Division responsible for the meeting (Medvedkov et al 1970) only received limited support: the Organization, committed as it was to the health and health service problems of rural areas, was not ready yet to recognize and respond to these emerging priorities. The results of a study undertaken in Cali, Colombia under this programme, correlating neighbourhood characteristics with infant and child mortality (Bertrand et al 1979), provides an idea of what was accomplished and continued to be accomplished by local researchers who went on applying the same methodology even without external support.

After the Alma Ata Conference in 1978, vulnerable and deprived urban groups received renewed attention. Urbanization and its health problems became more widely known and primary health care provided a multisectoral strategy that had a good chance of being effective to deal with them in the complex environment of the city. Thus, in 1983, a joint meeting of WHO and UNICEF on primary health care in urban areas proposed that the two organizations undertake the preparation of a State of the Art Report on the subject with special emphasis on the developing countries, slums and shanty areas and low income, deprived, at risk populations. The meeting concluded expressing

> *the conviction that the plight of those living in the slums and shanty towns of the developing world is one of the most important, yet least understood problems facing the human race. Many worthwhile projects are now in place, and there is an increasing fund of experience on which to draw. More people need to be aware of the scale and urgency of the problem, and of the approaches that should prove relevant, particularly those in position of leadership in the cities and countries of the developing world and in international organizations. Above all, more action is needed and rapid scaling up of current efforts from isolated institutions, until primary health care for people at risk in urban areas becomes a central component of national and international health care strategies.*
>
> (WHO/UNICEF 1983)

The requested State of the Art Report (WHO/UNICEF 1984a) was prepared as a collaborative effort of WHO and UNICEF and presented at a joint meeting in Guayaquil, Ecuador in 1984 (WHO/UNICEF 1984b). The intention of the report was to call attention to the magnitude of urbanization, its positive and negative features and its implications for health; to promote the cause of the urban poor; to stimulate awareness of the heterogeneity of the city and of the misleading way in which information about cities is analyzed and presented; to discuss the unique pattern of disease of the urban poor; to provide evidence that in comparing the health conditions of the poor in rural and in urban areas, the urban poor may be living in as severe and pressing conditions as those of the poor in rural areas; to criticize the lack of social relevance and equity in the way many urban health systems are organized; to discuss the organizational features of poor urban communities, their multiplicity and initial lack of structure if compared with most rural communities, but also their potential for action once they have organized themselves; to point to multisectoral action as the only way to approach the health problems of the urban poor; to describe initiatives that have attempted to improve the health conditions of the urban poor and to discuss constraints that have been met; to attempt a specification and synthesis of the qualities that urban health systems should have to fulfil their functions more equitably.

The Report was received with interest and referred to as 'a well argued and well disseminated paper that stimulated organizations to support preliminary research which explored what initiatives existed in urban health care and examined the nature of urban health problems' (Harpham and Stephens 1992). The content of the Report has subsequently been expanded and updated and developed into a book that was published in 1989 (Tabibzadeh et al 1989). A review published by the *Journal of Health Policy and Planning* included this book among the ten best readings in urban health planning (Stephens 1990).

At the WHO meeting in Quayaquil, where the State of the Art Report was presented, other important matters were discussed, namely the little awareness among the general public, even of the same cities, of the conditions in the 'misery belts' and the need, therefore, for consciousness raising initiatives; the need for continuing exchange of experience and the provision of backup support; the importance of the partnership between communities and public services as a *sine qua non* condition for primary health care and as something that can be achieved and sustained, but cannot be assumed; finally, the tough issue of scaling up beyond the project at local level and of changing the balance within the health care system to match the enormous rise of the current problem and to prepare for the continuing, explosive tempo of urbanization. Nobody, it was thought, can yet claim to have done this although some cities and countries had already made a brave start.

The Report was also used as the foundation for the formulation of the WHO programme of activities which is now being implemented. These activities went through different phases: initially, information and promotion predominated, followed by concern for technical development and the adaptation of the primary health care strategy to urban health development. At present, while activities in these areas continue and involve several programmes and divisions in WHO attention is increasingly given (also with the collaboration of Non-governmental organizations, cooperation agencies and research and development institutes) to providing support to specific initiatives and to reviewing and analyzing experiences and monitoring progress.

The Division of Strengthening of Health Services (SHS), initially responsible for initiating this process and the promotional activities summarized above, has specifically concentrated, as part of its wider mandate, on the development of health services in the urban areas of developing countries with emphasis on primary care and the poor.

In 1986, another joint Interregional Consultation was held in Manila (Philippines). Case studies were presented from cities in Bangladesh,

China, Colombia, Ethiopia, India, Indonesia, Republic of Korea, Mozambique, Nigeria, Pakistan, Philippines, Somalia, Sudan and Thailand and a rich experience reviewed. The consultation reiterated that primary health care is an appropriate strategy for achieving universal coverage on an equitable basis in urban areas, but also that the attention to the poor is insufficient and the reorientation of the health systems too slow a process. Matters such as referral, the involvement of agencies outside the health care sector and the various approaches to scaling up were considered and, in its conclusions, the consultation appealed to governments to promote and facilitate an early review of structures, facilities and methodologies available within countries for urban primary health care in order to determine the action steps that need to be taken, and to act urgently and decisively upon the findings. Intercity collaboration, within and between countries, was also recommended (WHO/UNICEF 1986).

In order to respond to the recommendations made at the various WHO meetings held so far, the Division of SHS formulated at this point a programme of activities that was published in 1988 (WHO 1988a), followed by a set of guidelines (WHO 1988b) for rapid appraisal to assess community health needs, intended for countries undertaking these kinds of investigations. A training workshop on health systems reorientation in urban areas to reach the underserved was also supported in Lusaka (Zambia) in April 1989 (WHO 1989).

Further review of developments was made at an interregional meeting on city health held in Karachi, Pakistan in 1989 (WHO 1990). The rationale behind organizing this meeting was the recognition that decision makers at city level have a key part to play in tackling the problems of the urban poor, although the constraints to which they are subjected are well recognized. There are a few recurring themes, understanding which, the meeting thought, 'may be the key to making the incomprehensible become clear, the overwhelming become manageable and the inevitable become avoidable' . These themes fall into the following four broad groups:

- the importance of understanding the scale of the problem;
- the location of responsibilities for health in the city;
- the importance of broader issues (particularly the interaction between urban and rural development) and their implications for city action; and
- the identification of means of addressing the health needs of the urban poor.

Allied to these themes are those of training, information and communication.

All these developments were a buildup to the 1991 World Health Assembly on urban health which is discussed in the next but one section.

URBAN ENVIRONMENTAL HEALTH

WHO is presently formulating and implementing a new global strategy on environmental health that places an important emphasis on urban health (WHO 1992b). In 1992, the United Nations Conference on Environment and Development (UNCED) adopted at the highest political level Agenda-21 – an action plan on environment and development to guide national and international action for the years to come (United Nations 1992). The global strategy is WHO's response to the programmes and responsibilities agreed upon by Member States at this Conference, and it provides the basis for WHO Headquarters, the Regional Offices and country programmes to develop workplans to implement Agenda-21. The work of the WHO Commission on Health and Environment has been central to the shaping of the health activities in Agenda-21 and in providing the basis for the new strategy. Highlights of the new strategy (WHO 1992b), as they apply to urban environmental health, are set out in the approaches and recommendations below (WHO 1992c) and one approach which is particularly important – the Healthy Cities Project – is also briefly described below.

Healthy Cities Project

The WHO Healthy Cities Project is best known for its work in cities throughout Europe, as well as the United States, Canada, Australia, New Zealand and Japan (WHO/EURO 1990). What is less well known is the rapid development of healthy cities projects in an increasing number of developing countries.

The objective of the Healthy Cities Project is to strengthen the capability and capacity of municipal governments, and to provide opportunities for individuals, families and community groups to deal with their health and environmental problems. 'Healthy Cities' achieves this by providing a framework that combines several key elements:

- increased awareness of health and environmental issues in urban development efforts by all municipal and national authorities;
- a network of cities that provides information exchange and technology transfer;
- a linkage of technical programmes for health and the environment with political mobilization and community participation. New partnerships are developed between municipal government agencies (health, water, sanitation, housing, social welfare etc), universities, NGOs, private companies and community organizations and groups to make the urban environment supportive of health rather than damaging to it.

Major developments in Healthy Cities in the early 1990s include:

In the **Eastern Mediterranean Region**, many countries are planning national networks of healthy cities. In Iran, a national meeting in Teheran was attended by 19 out of 23 of the provincial capital cities with 19 mayors in attendance and many key political figures. A healthy cities office has been set up in Teheran, and projects have been started to upgrade a number of low income housing areas in the city. In Pakistan, a national network of healthy cities has been established, and it is planned to commence projects in 12 major cities including all provincial capitals and the national capital. A number of other countries in the Region are setting up, or have plans to set up, similar networks including Saudi Arabia, Egypt, Yemen, Tunisia and Morocco. Many of the above cities participated in the Seventh International WHO Healthy Cities Symposium, Copenhagen, in 1992, with a particular interest in developing twinning arrangements with European cities.

In the **African Region**, in Ghana, the Accra Healthy Cities Project has undertaken a review of health problems in Accra, and is developing strategies and specific action plans to cover the following areas: environmental sanitation, food hygiene, development of urban health services, school health, public education and communication, community involvement in health and sanitation, and land use planning. The Ghanaian city of Kumasi is also participating. A series of further activities were identified with a particular focus on the role of subdistrict health management teams.

An African French-speaking network of healthy cities has been established, including Cameroon (Garoua), Chad (N'Djamena), Côte d'Ivoire (Abidjan, Toumodic), Gabon (Libreville), Niger (Niamey II, Dosso) and Senegal (Dakar, Rifisque, St Louis). The Third Global French-speaking Healthy Cities Congress took place in Montreal and Sherbrooke (Canada, Province of Quebec) in 1992, and cities located in all WHO Regions attended.

In the **Southeast Asia Region**, a network is being developed in six cities in various countries (Bangkok, Kanpur, Hyderabad, Dhaka, Surabaya, Colombo), and funding for initial activities is in the process of being secured. Healthy cities is a major focus of WHO intercountry activities on urban health in the Southeast Asia Regional Office.

In the **Americas** region, apart from Canada and the United States, healthy cities initiatives are in progress in Brazil (Rio de Janeiro), Bolivia and Colombia (in collaboration with Canada/Quebec). The Spanish Government, in collaboration with the Pan American Health Organization/WHO Regional Office for the Americas, is supporting a proposed network of healthy cities in Latin America. The WHO Collaborating Centre in Healthy Cities in Indiana is actively working to promote an international network of cities in this Region, and is also developing a global database on healthy cities.

In the **Western Pacific**, there have been discussions on a city networking project, 'healthy urban environments', that led to Healthy City Projects in China, Malaysia and Vietnam. Other projects have developed in Australia, New Zealand and Japan.

Recommendations for multilateral and bilateral support in urban environmental health

The following issues have been identified and elaborated by the WHO Commission (WHO 1992c) and are presented here as priority activities and/or recommendations:

1. There is a need for a **'foreign ministry' function of the health department**, to influence policies in other departments and agencies to incorporate health and environmental considerations into the

decision making process in industry, settlements planning, urban planning, municipal services etc. We have seen virtually all sectors of government and business have an important impact on urban health. The capacity of health departments must be enhanced to influence decision makers in all relevant sectors to consider the health impacts of their work.

2. **Environmental health** must be considered a high priority issue in large urban settings. Environmental health infrastructure is a cost-effective investment, given the cost (in lost exports, tourism, investment) of health disasters such as a cholera or meningitis epidemic to a city or country. Strengthening urban environmental health capabilities is essential, to support the provision of environmental services in water supply, sanitation, solid waste management and pollution control, and to allow use of health impact and environmental impact assessment procedures for urban development projects.

3. Recently, the identification and use of **intra-urban differences in health** has emerged as a key approach to draw public attention to problems, and to assist in mobilizing resources. To understand the environmental health problems in a city, information on health and environmental conditions must be geographically based so that differences between rich and poor neighbourhoods in the same city can be measured. City averages simply do not capture the urban reality. Very often health statistics related to poor areas are omitted or aggregated, and, therefore, hidden in the presentation of data from more privileged areas. Raising awareness and understanding is a vital prelude to action, and can be achieved through public education for health (in schools, the workplace, mass media etc) supported by documentation of intra-urban differences.

4. Traditional approaches to public health work in cities are no longer adequate. New **partnerships** must be developed between municipal government agencies (health, water, sanitation, housing, social welfare etc), universities, NGOs, private companies and community organizations and groups. The solutions to urban environmental health problems are to be found locally in strengthening existing, or developing new partnerships between municipal government and the local people and organizations, and decentralization of responsibilities to municipal government from the national level should be encouraged as far as is feasible. Strengthening of community participation in urban improvement activities can be achieved by the adoption of an 'enabling strategy' by the municipality, that emphasizes 'doing with' rather than 'doing for' (or providing services for).

5. Greater **coordination of urban development activities** by the various municipal government agencies can be assisted by development of a municipal health plan, including relevant social and environmental components, that involves: political commitment of the city to improved health and well being, and reduced inequalities in the city; building up of intersectoral committees at both the political and technical level; and establishing collaboration and links with

scientific, cultural, medical, business, social and other city institutions, using networking to gain political support and mobilize resources. These links can build a new sense of responsibility for health by the private sector, aided by government incentives. The plan must aim for 'sustainable' ecologically sound urban development, and planning processes that give incentives to consider health concerns in industrial, commercial, residential and infrastructure developments. It must be guided by an overall economic and fiscal framework which supports health and environment goals.

6. Establishment of **collaborative activities** and links with other cities (city networks), such as the WHO Healthy Cities programme, in order to exchange models of good practice. The benefits of networks of cities can be briefly stated:

   - Sharing of information and technologies between members.
   - Sharing of scarce resources to solve joint problems, eg, developing effective urban management strategies.
   - Joint development of standards or codes of good urban policies and management practices; the existence of such standards then has the effect of exerting pressure on all members of the network to adopt them, for no member wishes to become a bad example.
   - City networks have the potential to provide a force to influence national policies and norms to promote healthy urban development. This force can, for example, promote the decentralization of urban management functions and urban development decision making, from the national government level to the municipal government level, that is essential to allow local participation in urban development.

Some important research priorities identified by the Commission (WHO 1992b and 1992c) include:

- environmental health assessment monitoring – the environmental and health problems generated by rapid urbanization are not adequately reflected in current national or municipal statistics, because suitable indicators are not in use;
- community participation in the work of municipal agencies providing environmental services such as solid waste management, water, sanitation etc;
- evaluation and strengthening of programmes such as the WHO Healthy Cities programme which has been helpful in achieving public commitment by municipal governments, in establishing feasible health goals for cities, and in mobilizing the resources and participation of the community in pursuit of health;
- development and use of health impact and environmental impact assessment procedures for urban development projects.

WORLD HEALTH ASSEMBLY AND ITS FOLLOWUP

The importance and timeliness of the WHO concern for urban health development and the urban poor were underlined by the World Health Assembly decision to focus the Technical Discussions of its 44th session in May 1991 on 'Strategies for Health for All in the Face of Rapid Urbanization' (WHO 1991a). Working documents were prepared on a global overview on health and the cities, urban policies and health status, organization of urban health systems, development of urban environmental health services, cities and the population issue and city networks for health. These topics were discussed by the participants and the ensuing resolution (WHA 44.27) provides WHO with a renewed and explicit mandate to pursue its work in this area. The resolution specifically requested WHO to:

- strengthen its information base for the benefit of Member States and its own work in relation to the human and environmental aspects of urban development;
- strengthen its technical cooperation with countries in order to increase awareness of the needs of the urban poor, develop national skills to meet these needs and support the extension of city networks worldwide;
- promote regional networks and interdisciplinary panels of experts and community leaders, to advise on health aspects of urban development.

In encouraging participants to take a positive view and to identify opportunities for making a contribution to improving urban conditions and health, the Chairman of the Technical Discussions of the 44th World Health Assembly identified six personal imperatives:

1. To decentralize and put the emphasis for action at the municipal level.
2. To mobilize everyone who can help in city networks.
3. To invest in safe drinking water and waste disposal.
4. To help the poor to enhance their incomes and improve their housing.
5. To provide families with a range of sustainable health services in or near their homes with an emphasis on family planning as the centrepiece.
6. To ask the poor to identify their own needs and priorities and expect surprises.

In concurrence with the organization of the Technical Discussions of the Assembly, a corresponding issue of *World Health* (the magazine of WHO) was prepared and distributed under the title of 'Cities of Tomorrow' (WHO 1991b).

In response to the resolution of the 44th World Health Assembly, the Division of Strengthening of Health Services (SHS) undertook a series of initiatives. It coordinated, in collaboration with the Environmental Health Division, the preparation of an issue of the World Health Statistics Quarterly (Rossi-Espagnet et al 1991) with the participation of other technical programmes of WHO as an indication that the health and well being of the urban poor and the development of urban comprehensive health systems is a widespread responsibility in the Organization. The issue starts with an overall discussion of the urban crisis from various points of view and of the problems posed by the urban environment. It goes on to review the health effects of urbanization specifically focusing on problems of great present concern such as diet and nutrition, acute diarrhoeal diseases, acute respiratory infections, tuberculosis, meningitis, vaccine preventable diseases, malaria and other parasitic or arthropod transmitted diseases, sexually transmitted diseases including AIDS, zoonoses and mental conditions. It concludes with a discussion on the development and functioning of urban health systems based on current experiences and future perspectives.

SHS also convened a Study Group on Primary Health care in Urban Areas: The Role of Health Centres in the Development of Urban Health Systems (WHO 1992a). The Group reviewed the issues raised in the provision of ambulatory health services and the role of health centres in cities. The concept of 'reference health centres', based on recent experience, was put forward and the relationship was also considered of the peripheral health units with, on the one side, communities and individuals and, on the other side, hospitals of different levels through the referral process. Creative initiatives from Mexico City, Jakarta, Dar es Salaam, Bombay, Dakar, Los Angeles, São Paulo, Visakhapatnam and, in greater detail, from Cali, Manila and Newark were reported on and discussed. The problems of access and intersectoral backing seem to stand a good chance of being effectively tackled when there is a credible local facility with real roots in the community and good links to higher referral levels. Reference health centres, representing a useful and convenient blending of the roles and functions of hospitals and local health centres, seem to have potential as a method of improving urban health services. Their exact form will depend on local circumstances, but there should be a primary focus on what can be done locally with local and national resources and adequate attention paid to catchment areas, travel time and sound epidemiological understanding of the important local health problems. The group emphasized the need to increase the resources available to primary care. This could include the reallocation of resources to the periphery of the health system, the collection of user fees which remain under the budget of the health centre and the establishment of supportive links with Non-governmental organizations. The reference health centres, themselves, may result in increased resource generation because of the support they seem to enjoy from the communities they service (WHO 1992a).

In addition SHS developed other aspects of the health services that, although not specifically concerning low income urban populations, will contribute substantially to the improvement of the health services for the urban poor and advance their cause. Notable examples are the reorientation of the hospital system (WHO 1987), the development of health districts (Tarimo 1991), the financing of health services and the role and contributions of the private sector (WHO 1991c).

Finally, it initiated projects to promote development or improve the functioning of reference health centres in cities such as Bangkok, Calcutta,

Delhi, Jakarta, Harare, Madras and Manila. These projects are expected to contribute to improving the quality of care, expanding health care services to low income and underserved groups and establishing referral processes.

REGIONAL OFFICES

Along with developments at global level, matters related to urban health that is now an inter-regional project with Healthy City Units in each Regional Office that support regional networks of Healthy Cities.

Mention has already been made of the Healthy Cities Project developed under the auspices of the Regional Office for Europe, as it pertains to the European Region and also to other regions of WHO.

The Eastern Mediterranean Regional Office promoted a discussion on the implementation of primary health care and urban development was also considered (WHO/EMRO 1992).

A working group meeting was convened by the Western Pacific Regional Office in Osaka, Japan, in 1991. The group recognized that, while the health of the population was being undermined by shortcomings in the physical and social environment in practically all major cities of the region, the extent and impact of those shortcomings varied considerably between cities. Because of these differences and of those related to the level of resources, no common development model could be proposed. Rather, cities having different levels of development, problems and resources are being followed up and methods and approaches suitable to each will be identified and applied (WHO/WPRO 1991).

A corresponding initiative was taken by the SouthEast Asia Regional Office which in 1992 convened an intercountry consultation on health policies and strategies for urban slums. The objectives were to stimulate awareness and to support a conceptual and operational framework for both WHO/SEARO countries and to address the most urgent health needs of South East Asian cities in general and of their vast slum populations in particular.

Finally, the Pan American Health Organization (WHO Regional Office for the Americas) has frequently dealt with urban health in the context of its work on local health systems (PAHO 1990).

CONCLUSION

Urbanization has long been a concern of various international organizations, particularly those of the United Nations system such as FAO, HABITAT, ILO, UNDP and UNICEF. The World Bank has been particularly active in the area of urban infrastructure development and now sees urban health as an emerging priority (see Robert Hecht's chapter). WHO has monitored the health effects of urbanization and urban health development for many years. Its involvement has critically increased during the last decade. Activities went through different phases: initially, information and promotion predominated; this was followed by a period of concern for technical development and the application of the primary health care strategy to urban health development; at present, while activities in these areas continue and involve several programmes and divisions, attention is increasingly given (also with the collaboration of Non-governmental organizations and the support of cooperation agencies and research and development institutes) to providing support to specific developments, monitoring progress and reviewing and analyzing experiences. The Divisions of Environmental Health and Strengthening of Health Services, while continuing to devote attention to the health problems of rural areas, have been particularly active in urban health development. They have specifically concentrated on the development of health services in the urban areas of developing countries with emphasis on primary care and the poor, but have not neglected the health problems of urbanization in more industrialized societies. Numerous documents have been produced, some of which are mentioned in the list of references. A most notable event was the selection of the subject 'Strategies for health for all in the face of rapid urbanization' for the Technical Discussions of the 44th World Health Assembly in 1991 which provided WHO with a renewed and explicit mandate to pursue its work in this area (WHO 1991a). Specifically, WHO will:

- continue to pulicize the impending health crisis and encourage all those concerned to address the health problems of the urban poor;
- promote the reorientation of urban health systems towards primary health care: strengthened health departments and reference health centres, other health care units and public and private health institutions could play an important role in this transformation;
- continue to consider the development of a healthy and sustainable urban environment in urban settings of all sizes;
- identify and analyze examples of effective primary health care in urban areas and contribute to the development of methods to this effect;
- ensure the expansion and sustainability of successful schemes from their original area of development to all areas and populations for which they are ultimately intended;
- encourage and support economic studies of the impact on the financial and health costs, and benefits of reorienting urban health systems.

REFERENCES

Bertrand, W Blockett, P Levine, A (1979) A Methodology for Determining High Risk Components in Urban Environments *Int J Epidem*, 8, 2, pp161–66
Harpham, T and Stephens, C (1992) Policy Directions in Urban Health in Developing Countries – the Slum Improvement Approach *Social Science and Medicine*, 35, 2, pp111–120
Medvedkov, Y Myers, G Rossi-Espagnet, A (1970) A Programme for Ecological Studies of Urban Health Disorders, Division of Research in Epidemiology and Communication Science, WHO
Pan American Health Organization (1990) Development and Strengthening of Local Health Systems: Self-Evaluation of a Local System *Series Health Service Development* no 78
Pettersson, B et al (1992) *Playing for Time. Creating Supportive Environments for Health* Report from the Third International Conference on Health Promotion, Sundsvall, Sweden
Rossi-Espagnet, A Goldstein, G Abibzadeh, I (1991) Urbanization and Health in Developing Countries: A Challenge for Health for All *World Health Statistics Quarterly*, 44, 4, pp185–247

Stephens, C (1990) Ten Best Readings in... Urban Health Planning *Health Policy and Planning*, 5, 4, pp389–391

Tabibzadeh, I Rossi-Espagnet, A and Maxwell, R (1989) *Spotlight on the Cities: Improving Urban Health in Developing Countries*, WHO, Geneva

Tarimo, E (1991) *Towards a Healthy District. Organizing and Managing District Health Systems Based on Primary Health care*, WHO, Geneva

United Nations (1992) Conference on Environment and Development, Rio de Janeiro, 1–12 June 1992

World Health Organization (1963) Urban Health Services. Fifth Report of the Expert Committee on Public Health Administration *WHO Technical Report Series* no 250, Geneva

World Health Organization (1970) Report of the Meeting on the Health Effects of Urbanization, Geneva, 2– 7 November (unpublished document)

World Health Organization (1987) Hospitals and Health for All: Report of a WHO Expert Committee on the Role of Hospitals at the First Referral Level *WHO Technical Report Series*, no 744

World Health Organization (1988a) *Improving Urban Health: A Programme for Action* Geneva, Division of Strengthening of Health Services (unpublished document WHO/SHS/NHP/88.2)

World Health Organization (1988b) *Improving Urban Health: Guidelines for Rapid Appraisal to Assess Community Health Needs* (unpublished document WHO/SHS/NHP/88.4)

World Health Organization (1989) *Training Workshop on Health System Reorientation in Urban Areas to Reach the Underserved; Learning Material to Assess and Plan, Lusaka (Zambia), 17–27 April 1989* (unpublished document WHO/SHS/NHP/89.4)

World Health Organization (1990) *Report of the Interregional Meeting on City Health: The Challenge of Social Justice, Karachi (Pakistan), 27–30 November 1989* (unpublished document WHO/SHS/NHP/90.3)

World Health Organization (1991a) 44th World Health Assembly *Report of Technical Discussions, Strategies for Health for All in the Face of Rapid Urbanization* (unpublished WHO document A44/Technical Discussions/8, 14 May 1991)

World Health Organization (1991b) *World Health* Cities of Tomorrow, March–April

World Health Organization (1991c) *Report of an Interregional Meeting on the Public/Private Mix in National Health Systems and the Role of Ministries of Health, Hacienda Cocoyoc, State of Morelos, Mexico, 22–26 July 1991* (unpublished document WHO/SHS/NHP/91.2)

World Health Organization (1992a) The Role of Health Centres in the Development of Urban Health Systems, Report of a WHO Study Group on Primary Health care in Urban Areas *WHO Technical Report Series*, no 827

World Health Organization (1992b) *Our Planet, Our Health* Report of the WHO Commission on Health and Environment

World Health Organization (1992c) *Report on Urbanization* WHO Commission on Health and Environment

World Health Organization Regional Office for the Eastern Mediterranean (1992) Followup meeting for PHC directions on PHC implementation, Cairo, 22–27 February

World Health Organization Regional Office for Europe (1990) Tsouros, A (ed) *Healthy Cities Project: A Project Becomes a Movement, Review of Progress 1987 to 1990*

World Health Organization Regional Office for South East Asia (1992) *Report of the Intercountry Consultation on Health Policies and Strategies for Urban Slums, New Delhi, 3–7 August 1992*

World Health Organization Regional Office for the Western Pacific (1991) *Report of the Regional Working Group on Urban Health Development in the Western Pacific Region, Osaka (Japan), 18–21 September 1991* (Report Series no RS/91/GE/18/JPN))

World Health Organization/United Nations Childrens Fund (1983) *Report of the UNICEF-WHO Meeting on Primary Health care in Urban Areas, Geneva, 23–29 July 1983* (unpublished WHO document SHS/HSR/83.1)

World Health Organization/United Nations Childrens Fund (1984a) *Primary Health care in Urban Areas: Reaching the Urban Poor in Developing Countries. A State of the Art Report*, Geneva (prepared by Rossi-Espagnet, A)

World Health Organization/United Nations Childrens Fund (1984b) *Joint UNICEF-WHO Consultation on Primary Health care in Urban Areas, Guayaquil (Ecuador), 15–19 October 1984* (unpublished WHO document SHS/84.5)

World Health Organization/United Nations Childrens Fund (1986) *Interregional Consultation on Primary Health care in Urban Areas, Manila (Philippines), 7–11 July 1986* (unpublished WHO document SHS/IHS/86.1)

8

Urban Health – an Emerging Priority for the World Bank

Robert Hecht

INTRODUCTION

In the years that have followed the major internal reorganization of the World Bank in the late 1980s, lending and related analytical activities in the areas of health, population and nutrition have increased dramatically. Within this domain, urban health is now emerging as an important new priority for Bank support.

This chapter documents the recent rise in World Bank assistance for health in developing countries and the emergence of urban health as an important theme. It explains the intellectual and political origins of this shift. And it examines the different types of World Bank assistance for urban health programme and policy reforms. It argues that urban health can be expected to remain a central focus of the Bank's work in the health sector for the rest of the 1990s. This is because of the growing concentration of the developing world's poor in urban areas, and because improving the efficiency of urban based hospitals is an essential ingredient in national health sector reform.

THE ASCENDANCE OF HEALTH IN THE WORLD BANK'S PORTFOLIO

Compared with other sectors such as agriculture and power generation, the complex of health, population, and nutrition is a relatively new area for the World Bank. Lending for these activities only began in the 1970s, more than 25 years after the Bank was founded as part of the Bretton Woods agreements. The early Bank projects of the 1970s were mainly entirely related to population and typically included support for the development of national population policies and for the expansion of family planning services. The first Bank-financed health project per se was only approved in 1976, and the Bank's first major health policy statement was published in 1980. During 1980–1982, the Bank approved just seven new projects in health and population, or an average of just over two a year.

There was a dramatic increase in Bank support for health, however, in the second half of the 1980s. The number of new projects approved annually rose from an average of eight in 1987–1989 to 21 in 1990–1992 (Figure 8.1), and the value of credits and loans committed grew from an average of $317 million to $1151 million over the same period (Figure 8.2). As a share of new World Bank lending, projects for health, population and nutrition increased from less than 1 per cent in 1987 to nearly 7 per cent in 1992.

Based only on projects which have already been approved, World Bank disbursements for health rose from about $300 million in 1992 to $1000 million in 1995. To put this in perspective, this anticipated level of spending is equivalent to over 20 per cent of the $4800 million in total external assistance for health in developing countries in 1990. Disbursements of $1000 million annually would make the World Bank by far the largest source of aid to the health sector, well ahead of USAID, which was the leading donor with disbursements of $585 million in 1990.

The upsurge in Bank lending for health, population and nutrition has been strongly underpinned by a concomitant rise in the volume of analytical work on health issues in developing countries. The average number of country specific studies of health issues grew from 16 in 1984–1986 to 18 in 1987–1989 and 30 in 1990–1992. This growth has been accompanied by a diversification in the topics covered, away from broadbrush sector surveys to more indepth analyses of problems of health financing, AIDS, epidemiological change and health service organization and management.

The rapid expansion of World Bank analyses of health issues and of technical and financial assistance for health in the late 1980s was stimulated by a renewed Bank commitment to human resources

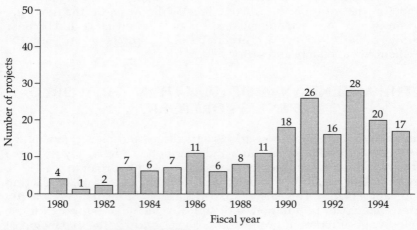

Source: Annual Operational Review, 1992 (PHN)

Figure 8.1 *Lending for the population, health and nutrition sector, 1980–1995 Number of projects*

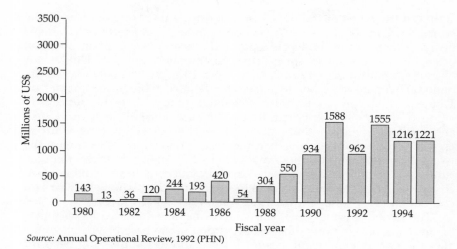

Source: Annual Operational Review, 1992 (PHN)

Figure 8.2 *Lending for the population, health and nutrition sector, 1980–1995 Commitments to PHN and Social Development Projects*

development in general. This commitment spanned the entire institution and was articulated by senior Bank officials including Barber Conable when he took over as President in 1987. Conable pledged major increases in Bank lending for population, nutrition and food security, basic education and women in development, as well as health.

Bank emphasis on human resources has been strongly reinforced by a parallel concern to make the alleviation of poverty the primary goal of the institution. The 1990 *World Development Report* (World Bank 1990b) was devoted to the topic of poverty and policies for its reduction; a policy statement on the Bank's role in poverty alleviation and a *Poverty Reduction Handbook* (World Bank 1992c) containing guidelines and practical examples of countrywide poverty assessments and poverty reduction projects followed in 1991 and 1992. These documents emphasize the importance of investing in basic health services, especially low cost preventive care, as a way of mitigating poverty. Better health for the poor is seen as a means to enhancing their productivity and incomes, improving the educability of their children, and generally improving their well being.

URBAN HEALTH – AN EMERGING THEME FOR THE WORLD BANK

The rationale for Bank involvement in urban health

In the last several years, health policies and programmes in the urban milieu have become an important emerging theme in the World Bank's work in the health sector in developing countries. There are two main reasons for this. First, poverty is widespread in urban areas – investing in health for the poor means in part improving health services and health status in the cities of the developing world. About one quarter of the world's urban dwellers – 325 million people – live in poverty. This is nearly 30 per cent of the world's poor. The health of the urban poor can often be worse than in rural areas; in the slum areas of Dhaka, for example, infant mortality rates of 134 per 1000 births easily exceed the national average of 94 per 1000 (see the detailed table in the chapter by Tanner and Harpham). Data from Demographic and Health Surveys in eight countries – Brazil, Egypt, Kenya, Nigeria, Peru, Senegal, Sri Lanka and Thailand – suggest that while average child mortality rates in urban areas are consistently lower than the corresponding rural averages, the worst off urban communities have higher child mortality levels than the rural average. In Brazil and Thailand, child mortality in some poor urban clusters is twice the rural average (background calculations by Ken Hill and Barbara McKinney for the 1993 *World Development Report*).

The second reason for the Bank's increasing attention to urban health is the growing recognition of the importance of urban based hospitals in the allocation of national resources for health, and of the pressing need for hospital reforms as part of broader policy changes in the health sector. Studies of health expenditure in developing countries show that a minimum of 40 per cent of government health budgets, and sometimes as much as 80 per cent , is spent on hospitals (World Bank 1993). A single large tertiary care facility in the capital or other urban centre, often linked to a medical school, can absorb a sizeable share of public expenditures for health. The University Teaching Hospital in Lusaka, Zambia, consumes 15 per cent of the Ministry of Health budget; Kenyatta National Hospital in Nairobi uses over 10 per cent of the Kenyan government's allocation for health (World Bank 1991); and the four central hospitals in Harare and Bulawayo account for a quarter of the health budget in Zimbabwe (World Bank 1992d).

Recent analysis also reveals that a sizeable share of government subsidies to these hospitals benefits the middle class and the wealthy and that an important part of hospital expenditure is simply wasted. In Lesotho, for example, an assessment of spending by the national referral hospital in Maseru, the capital, found considerable wastage on drugs and supplies by specifically identified hospital departments. The savings on drugs alone from improved selection, procurement, cost accounting, prescribing and dispensing was estimated at 10 to 20 per cent of the hospital budget for pharmaceuticals (background study by W Bicknell 1990).

The analytical foundations for Bank action

A growing body of analysis of urban health issues by World Bank staff and consultants, complementing the much larger efforts of other researchers and development institutions, has underpinned the Bank's movement towards policy reform and programme lending for urban health. There are several strands to this analytical work. A first is the series of studies of the changing epidemiological profile, health needs and related health priorities of such developing countries as China and Brazil (World Bank 1992a, World Bank 1990a). In the Brazil study, the enormous intra-urban differences in health status between wealthy and poor households were noted for a number of cities. In Porto Alegre, for example, infant mortality of 43 per 1000 births among the poor was more than twice the rate of 19 per 1000 for the rich. Similarly, male adult mortality for the poor of 1800 per 100,000 annually was about 50 per cent higher than for the wealthy.

The second strand involves a number of sponsored household surveys by the Bank that reveal major problems of access to basic public health services and to clinical care in primary facilities and at first level referral hospitals. These surveys, carried out under the Living Standards Measurement Surveys and Social Dimensions of Adjustment programme, show that the poor have to travel greater distances and wait longer to receive services which are often of inferior quality. While restricted access to basic services for the poor is especially critical in the rural areas of countries such as Peru and Côte d'Ivoire (World Bank 1993), it is also a problem in urban areas.

The third strand of analytical work deals with hospitals, especially government hospitals: their preponderant weight in public spending for health and relatively modest benefits in terms of health gains; and their pervasive inefficiencies and possible steps to improve hospital efficiency. A major study of hospitals in developing countries undertaken by Barnum and Kutzin (1993) documents the major share of public resources devoted to hospitals; articulates a methodology for assessing hospital efficiency; and points to sources of inefficiency and ways to reduce waste (Box 8.1). The book draws upon a wide range of World Bank and other studies of individual countries and individual hospitals, including Bank sector reports on China, Nigeria, Turkey and Zimbabwe, and a large number of broad reviews of public expenditure carried out routinely by the Bank to strengthen its dialogue with developing countries on macro-economic issues.

The study by Barnum and Kutzin argues that the medical conditions that occur with the greatest frequency in the population can be treated in relatively simple facilities, while truly severe conditions requiring sophisticated tertiary care occur relatively infrequently. In a well functioning national hospital system, therefore, district hospitals would have the highest turnover rates and tertiary hospitals the lowest. Similarly, because length of stay is generally greater for patients with more severe and complex conditions, tertiary hospitals would have the longest stays and district hospitals the shortest. However, as shown in Table 8.1, the experience of many countries does not follow this pattern. Some countries such as China and Fiji are efficient: tertiary hospitals have the longest stays and lowest turnover rate, and district hospitals have the lowest stays and highest turnover. In Papua New Guinea, however, the low turnover rate for district hospitals implies that there is relatively little demand for care at this level, a situation which may result because district hospitals have too many beds relative to the population they serve or the services may be of such poor quality that patients bypass them for higher levels. The shorter average stays at the tertiary hospital suggests that many patients not requiring tertiary care are treated at this hospital, possibly due to a lack of viable district hospital alternatives for the low income urban population or bypassing of lower level facilities because of poor quality.

Box 8.1

ASSESSING HOSPITAL PERFORMANCE IN INDONESIA

Cost studies can be supplemented by examination of service statistics to rapidly identify hospitals in developing countries with substandard inpatient performance. Once the hospitals are identified, analysis of specific efficiency issues can move beyond the realm of economics and into management, organization and personnel planning.

It is hard to make absolute statements about hospital efficiency from unit cost data, because of differences in quality of care and case mix across hospitals: higher unit costs at one facility relative to another may reflect higher quality, poorer efficiency, a more severely ill mix of patients or a combination of these factors. However, there are some fairly easy to use tools available to assess hospital performance relative to other hospitals within a country. These are inpatient service statistics: the bed turnover rate (inpatients per bed per year), average length of patient stay (ALOS) and the bed occupancy rate (percentage of total hospital beds occupied).

If treatment costs are similar in two hospitals, higher occupancy rates in one tend to result in lower average costs per patient day because overhead costs are spread over beds that are usually filled. However, if high occupancy results from relatively few admissions with a very long ALOS, hotel and overhead costs will be high relative to the number of patients and average cost per inpatient admission will be high. The expected marginal cost per patient day would be low because the treatment costs at the end of a long hospital stay tend to be minimal. Alternatively, if the bed turnover rate is high, average cost per inpatient is apt to be lower because hotel costs are spread over a larger number of patients, whereas the marginal cost per day would be relatively high. Increasing the bed occupancy rate via a greater number of admissions per bed rather than by increasing ALOS allows more patients to be served and thus improves hospital productivity.

Each of the three inpatient service indicators – ALOS, bed occupancy and bed turnover rates – is usually defined on an annual basis and can refer to a particular ward, inpatient department, entire hospital or group of hospitals. Any one of these indicators provides useful information which can help describe the performance of a hospital's inpatient services, but their explanatory power is multiplied when they are used together. Because they are mathematically interrelated, knowledge of any two indicators defines the third. The graphical approach developed for Colombian hospitals by Pabón Lasso (1986) uses the indicators together to enable rapid identification of hospitals that exhibit signs of technical inefficiency. It is applied here to Indonesia.

Each point in the figure in this Box represents one of 78 Indonesian Type C (district level) hospitals (18 on Sumatra, 43 on Java and 17 on the other islands). The points are defined by the bed turnover and occupancy rates for each hospital, which in turn define the ALOS. Because of the mathematical relationship among these three indicators of hospital performance, a ray drawn from the origin which passes through any point on the graph represents a constant average length of stay. The dotted lines are one standard deviation (plus and minus) from the means of the occupancy and turnover rates. Hospitals which lie outside the central rectangle formed by the intersecting dotted lines are considered outliers and merit further investigation to understand their deviation from the norm.

Hospitals in region I exhibit excess bed availability, low demand relative to installed capacity, and possibly demand which has been reduced by the diversion of patients to competing facilities. Region II is characterized by excess bed availability, unnecessary hospitalizations or the use of beds for patient observation (leading to a high proportion of very short stays), and a predominance of normal (as opposed to complicated) deliveries. Hospitals in region III are the relatively good performers, as evidenced by both their high turnover rates and moderate ALOS, suggesting a relatively small proportion of unused capacity. Hospitals in region IV may have one or all of the following: a high proportion of severe patients, predominance of chronic cases and unnecessarily long inpatient stays.

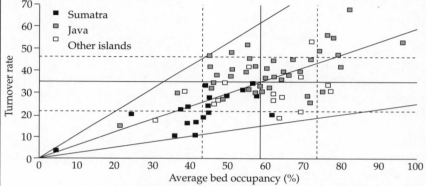

Indicators of hospital performance, Indonesia, Type C hospitals, 1985

The graph highlights the apparently poor performance of hospitals in Sumatra (concentrated in Region I), as compared to those of Java and the other islands. This region is characterized by low demand for hospital beds relative to installed capacity, either because of a generalized low demand for inpatient care or because alternatives to Type C beds are preferred by the population. Under these circumstances, it might be cost effective to consolidate inpatient services in a smaller number of facilities and to convert some facilities into strictly ambulatory centres. This would enable reallocation of staff and allow remaining Type C facilities to become more productive. If demand for inpatient care at a Type C hospital is low because the population bypasses this hospital to reach a higher level hospital, it might be appropriate to improve the quality of services at the Type C hospital (for example by transferring physicians from higher level hospitals to the Type C) in order to change the population's preferences and improve the referral system. Alternatively, if this is not feasible, it might be better to curtail the inpatient services of the Type C hospital, by closing hospitals or scaling them back.

Sources: Barnum, Howard. 'Hospital Expenditure in Indonesia.' PHN Technical Note 87-17. Population, Health and Nutrition Department, World Bank, Washington, DC

Barnum, Howard and Joseph Kutzin 1993 *Public Hospitals in Developing Countries: Resource Use, Cost, Financing*. Baltimore: Johns Hopkins University Press for the World Bank.

Pabón Lasso, Hipolito 1986 'Evaluating Hospital Performance through Simultaneous Application of Several Indicators.' *Bulletin of the Pan American Health Organization* 20(4):341-357.

Table 8.1 *Hospital service statistics, selected countries*

Country and year of data	Level of hospital	Occupancy rate (%)	Bed turn-over rate per year	Average length of stay	No. of hospitals in study
Belize (1985)	Central	68	40.7	6.1	1
	District	31	37.3	3.0	6
China (1986)	Tertiary	94	13.7	25.1	8
	Provincial	86	17.6	17.9	11
	District	95	26.1	13.3	7
Ethiopia	Urban	47	14.7	11.8	6
(1983–1985)	Rural	59	29.7	7.2	13
Fiji (1987)	Tertiary	83	42.5	7.2	3
	District	46	47.9	3.5	19
Indonesia	Tertiary	75	29.2	9.4	2
(1985)	Provincial	68	28.7	8.7	15
	District	54	33.6	5.9	296
Jamaica	Tertiary	79	35.2	8.2	5
(1985)	Mid-level	84	43.2	7.1	4
	District	61	28.6	7.8	13
Lesotho	Central	125	50.7	9.0	1
(1985)	District	129	54.9	8.6	7
Papua New	Tertiary	80	29.4	9.9	1
Guinea	Regional	80	28.1	10.4	4
(1988)	District	60	16.9	12.9	8
Zimbabwe	Central	89	41.7	7.8	4
(1987)	Provincial	91	54.5	6.1	8
	District	76	40.8	6.8	31

Source: Adapted from Barnum and Kutzin (1993)

Lending for urban health

A sizeable proportion of recent World Bank health projects that now focus exclusively on urban health, or have a major urban health component, as shown in Table 8.2. All nine urban oriented projects identified, with a total estimated cost of $489.5 million and World Bank financing of $353.1 million (72 per cent of the total) are currently under implementation. The nine projects are spread over virtually all of the major developing regions: three in Africa, three in Asia, two in Latin America and one in the Middle East. Both the newness and geographical diversity of these projects point to the very recent emergence of urban health as a major theme in World Bank lending.

The new urban health projects generally follow one of two main approaches that grow out of the twin concerns of the Bank for urban poverty and for hospital efficiency. The Bolivia integrated health project, the two India family welfare projects and the Philippines health and nutrition operation concentrate squarely on improving access to and quality of basic health services for the urban poor. They do so by targeting

Box 8.2

IMPROVING FAMILY WELFARE SERVICES IN BOMBAY AND MADRAS

Background The level of urbanization in India since Independence is low relative to other developing countries, but this situation is changing rapidly. The urban population is expected to double to at least 320 million in 2000, or about 30 per cent of the national total. The bulk of the migrants to India's major cities become slum dwellers and their demographic characteristics are not known with any precision. However, while urban birth and death rates are in general lower than rural rates, they mask wide differentials between the more affluent middle and upper classes and slum dwellers. Most poor people live without sanitation or potable water, in crowded, unventilated slum shacks, conditions that are conducive to high morbidity and mortality rates, particularly for young children.

Although Bombay has the most diversified economy of India's major cities, as well as higher than average income levels, conditions are appalling in its extensive slum areas, including some 400,000 persons who live in 20,000 deteriorating tenements in the southern part of Bombay Island and about 200,000 pavement dwellers.

Madras is India's fourth largest city. The population now included in the Madras City Municipal Corporation has grown rapidly over the last four decades, from 0.9 million in 1941 to 3.3 million in 1981, and is estimated to have reached about 4 million by 1987. The slum population is estimated to be about 1.6 million or 40 per cent of the total.

Goals and Objectives The principal goal of the $78.2 million project is to assist in the implementation of the Indian government's policies and programmes for revamping the organizational, service delivery, and outreach systems for family welfare in urban slums and congested areas, as part of the national Urban Revamping Scheme.

The specific objectives of the project are to: (1) expand family welfare services with the emphasis on maternal and child health, birth spacing and increased use of temporary contraceptive methods in the Greater Bombay, Madras City and the Chingleput district in Tamil Nadu; (2) improve the quality of family welfare services delivered in these urban areas; (3) strengthen the capacity of Tamil Nadu, Bombay and Madras to plan, manage, and implement family welfare programme in urban areas; and (4) increase the participation of private voluntary organizations (PVOs) and private medical practitioners (PMPs) in the urban family welfare programme.

Project Activities The service delivery expansion objective is being achieved by building, furnishing, equipping and staffing of new health posts and the rehabilitation/extension of existing health facilities. The quality improvement objective is being achieved by the training of all categories of family welfare workers in both cities. The management improvement objective is being pursued in Bombay by creating a Central Coordinating Office in the public health department and three Family Welfare Bureaus; and in Tamil Nadu by strengthening the State and Madras City Family Welfare Bureaus. The objective of increasing PVO and PMP participation in the family welfare programme in Bombay, Madras and Chingleput is being accomplished by assisting PVOs to operate health posts, devolving health worker training and selected information/education activities to PVOs, supporting innovative schemes of PVOs, and providing upgrading training and supplies to PMPs.

Overall, the project is attempting to increase the number of urban health posts from 56 to 195 in Bombay and from 45 to 152 in Madras; to boost effective contraceptive prevalence from 25 to 60 per cent; increasing immunization coverage from 55 to 95 per cent; and reach 95 per cent of all pregnant women with antenatal and postnatal care.

Benefits The proposed project is directly benefiting low income families, particularly about 1.6 million women and about 0.9 million children. Wider acceptance of family planning can have important benefits for the health of both mothers and children. Increasing the birth spacing interval can significantly decrease infant mortality because mothers are stronger during pregnancy and lactation and infants are born with higher birthweights. Priority interventions including antenatal care, identification of high risk pregnancies, institutional delivery for all pregnancies and immunization should have a significant impact on mother and child survival. Other large Indian cities facing the same service delivery constraints will be well-served by the experiences of this project. Designed to deliver a manageable package of family welfare interventions in poor communities and meet priority needs, the project is developing outreach, management, and supervision systems which could be models elsewhere. Forging an effective collaborative partnership with PVOs to share community responsibilities and undertaking to strengthen other private sector contributions to family welfare targets should provide valuable experience in effective government/private sector collaboration.

Box 8.3

INCREASING HOSPITAL EFFICIENCY IN NAIROBI, KENYA

Background Over the past 25 years, Kenya has made substantial progress in improving the overall health of its population. Health indicators have progressed steadily and are considerably better than those of most countries at similar levels of development. Since independence in 1963, life expectancy has risen from 42 to 58 years, and under five mortality has correspondingly declined from 200 to 110 per 1000 live births. This progress is due in large part to the rapid expansion of government financed programmes during the 1960s and 1970s.

During the 1980s, as rising demand from Kenya's rapidly growing population and the need for fiscal restraint imposed severe constraints on the Government's ability to finance expansion into underserved areas, expansion was curtailed and the quality of existing government services declined. Efforts to restrain the growth of expenditure fell heavily on drugs, consumables, equipment and maintenance, while personnel costs continued to rise. In addition, a large and growing share of public spending on health was devoted to urban hospitals, reflecting their high costs and minimal cost recovery, further limiting the scope for expanding services and for more cost-effective preventive and primary health programmes, especially in rural areas.

The present referral system within the public subsector allows patients to move from the primary to the tertiary level without effective control by medical professionals. The lack of any demand allocation mechanism, combined with the widespread and largely accurate perception that the quality of care is better at the higher levels of the health system, has led to patients bypassing facilities and going directly to district and provincial hospitals, including Kenyatta National Hospital (KNH). The result has been overcrowding and inefficient use of hospitals. The charging system, referral policy and most importantly, improved quality and availability of primary care are key to reversing this situation. Some health centres and dispensaries, on the other hand, are underutilized or idle because of a lack of personnel, diagnostic equipment, drugs and other medical supplies, or because a large proportion of the medical equipment is not functioning due to lack of spare parts, repairs and maintenance. These problems are particularly pronounced in the Nairobi area.

Objectives The project's main objective is to support the government's programme of health sector reform by (1) rehabilitating KNH to reduce its burden on the overall budget and permit an increase in expenditure on preventive and primary health; (2) improving the delivery of health services in the Nairobi area; and (3) preparing for future policy, managerial and investment reform in health.

The project, designed to be implemented over a four year period from 1991, includes the following major components:

Kenyatta National Hospital (US$20.7 million base cost), including its physical rehabilitation and institutional development. Project elements include (1) civil works to upgrade and rehabilitate existing buildings and facilities; (2) medical and non-medical equipment, beds and vehicles; (3) HIV/AIDS-related supplies; (4) training of managers and technicians; and (5) technical assistance and computers to strengthen the management of finance, personnel, and procurement.

Nairobi Area Health Services (US$4.4 million base cost) including interim improvements in service delivery, developing a strategic health plan for the Nairobi area, and modest funding of its initial implementation. Project elements include (1) technical assistance to develop a strategic plan; and (2) rehabilitation and construction, equipment, training, and technical assistance to meet priority needs at selected Nairobi City Commission and Ministry of Health facilities.

Strengthening Health Planning and Analysis and Preparing Sector Reform (US$3.3 million base cost), including strengthening the capacity of the Divisions of Planning and Development and of Family Health in the Ministry of Health, a series of analytical studies of the health sector, establishing a public investment programme for health, and developing a phased programme of sectoral reform. Project elements include (1) technical assistance, staff training, computers and office equipment for the Division of Planning and Development; and (2) analytical studies and technical assistance to prepare a reform programme and a public investment programme for the health sector.

Benefits The project will improve the allocation and mobilization of resources in the health sector in Kenya. Resource allocation improvements will result from all three health components. The KNH component will rehabilitate and improve the efficiency of the hospital, making it financially viable. Fees as a proportion of its spending will rise from 2 per cent in 1989/1990 to 23 per cent by 1995/1996 and its average length of inpatient stay will drop from 8.6 to 7.1 days over the same period. This will set an important example for the rest of the curative health system, which could lead to further efficiency improvements at other hospitals in the future. By reducing KNH's burden on the government's recurrent budget for health from 14 to 12 per cent, the KNH component will also permit an increased allocation of resources to preventive and primary services, on which returns are highest. By starting the process of rationalizing health care in the Nairobi area, the second project component will also improve the allocation of resources and of demand in the city; the strategic plan to be developed will provide a framework for rational investment programming in Nairobi.

Table 8.2 *World Bank lending for urban health*

Country and project	Implementation period	Total estimated cost ($ million)	World Bank financing ($ million)	Main urban health objectives
Bolivia: Integrated health development	1991–1996	38.6	20.0	Improve maternal and child health status in the poor urban and peri-urban areas of the country's four largest cities.
Chile: Technical assistance and hospital rehabilitation	1993–1996	45.3	27.0	Enhance the quality of hospital services in six health service areas in the poor urban and semi-urban communities of Santiago.
India: Fifth population (Bombay and Madras)	1988–1995	78.2	57.0	Improve availability and quality of family welfare services (family planning, maternity care, immunizations) in urban slums of Bombay and Madras, through construction and renovation of facilities, development of outreach programmes, and increased participation by private organizations.
India: Family welfare (urban slums)	1993–2000	96.6	79.0	Increase the supply, quality and demand for family welfare services in slum areas of Bangalore, Calcutta, Delhi and Hyderabad.
Kenya: Hospital rehabilitation	1992–1997	34.5	31.0	Rehabilitate Kenyatta National Hospital in order to improve its internal efficiency and its delivery of primary care; and expand clinical services in the Nairobi area.
Lesotho: Second health, population and nutrition	1991–1996	21.5	12.1	Improve efficiency and quality of health services at the central hospital, by reducing referrals and bypassing urban primary care centres in poor neighbourhoods and by developing better management systems.

Project	Period			Objectives
Mozambique: Health and nutrition	1990–1995	42.5	27.0	Raise quality and efficiency of health services, by reconstructing selected urban facilities, strengthening hospital management and developing maintenance programmes.
Philippines: Urban health and nutrition	1994–2001	82.8	70.0	Reduce urban poverty by improving health and nutrition service availability and quality in slums of Manila, Cebu and Cagayan de Oro; by building the capacity of city and municipal governments to plan and manage health programmes; and by developing cost-effective urban outreach activities.
Tunisia: Hospital restructuring support	1992–1997	49.5	30.0	Improve hospital efficiency and financing by developing management skills and systems, reorganizing administrative units and upgrading equipment and facilities.

Box 8.4

RATIONALIZING URBAN HEALTH SERVICES IN MASERU, LESOTHO

Background The Ministry of Health in 1980 introduced an integrated system for delivering health services in Lesotho, with three basic layers of institutions and personnel: (1) at village level, a network of 4000 volunteer village health workers, supported by the Village Development Councils; (2) above the village, a series of clinics or health centres, each with a catchment population of 6000 to 10,000 persons; and (3) above the clinic, by the 18 Health Service Areas (HSA) which cover the entire country, each with its general hospital as the first line of referral and its own health team liaising with the District Development Committee. The Ministry operates nine general hospitals with a total of 1137 beds, including Queen Elizabeth II Hospital (QE II) in Maseru, which also serves as the national referral hospital. The Ministry also runs two specialized hospitals for mental health and leprosy. Church missions own and run the other nine hospitals in the country, each one overseeing an HSA.

Current patterns of facility use are uneven, with some church hospitals operating at well below capacity, while QE II and some district hospitals are severely overcrowded. The hospitals are especially overburdened by outpatients seeking treatment for relatively minor ailments and by routine maternity cases that could be treated more cost-effectively in clinics. This is caused by lack of coordination between the Ministry and the missions in planning and fee-setting, inadequate incentives and procedures for patient referral and insufficient staffing of peripheral facilities. To improve this situation, urban filter clinics were established under the first World Bank-assisted project (1984–1990) in Maseru, Leribe and Mafeteng, and a fee differential between hospitals and clinics was introduced in July 1988.

While QE II faces the same overcrowding and quality of service issues as other facilities, its difficulties are magnified by the hospital's size (450 beds), budget (40 per cent of recurrent health spending), and multiple functions as neighbourhood clinic for Maseru, district hospital for Maseru HSA, and referral hospital for the country. A 1988 study of the facility identified the following key weaknesses: extreme overcrowding of wards; poor physical condition of buildings; shortages of basic equipment; lack of maintenance capability; uneven distribution of workload; weak planning, staff development and supervision, and financial management. A major programme to upgrade the hospital's physical plant and improve its organization and management formulated in the study is being implemented under the present project.

Objective The project objectives include strengthening the decentralized health service infrastructure and logistical support system, both in rural and urban areas, and improving the efficiency of service delivery. In order to achieve this objective, the project supports expansion of urban health services through upgrading of QE II Hospital (civil works, equipment, training and technical assistance) and development of urban filter clinics.

To shift some of the existing patient load away from the hospitals, the Ministry has decided that further changes in the hierarchy of urban health facilities are required. It is proposing to establish in a phased manner a series of urban 'filter' clinics (FC) that would be distinguished from community clinics by their larger size and nursing staff, around the clock service, on-site staff accommodation and assignment of a doctor on a full or half time basis. Five ordinary community clinics would be linked to one FC, with referrals from clinic to FC and ultimately to a hospital. An FC would thus have a catchment population of 25,000–50,000. To perform its assigned function, it would concentrate on providing outpatient care and routine emergency and maternity services.

Project activities To help initiate this programme to improve the quality and accessibility of urban health services and promote decongestion of QE II Hospital, the project would support the creation of three FC in Maseru and one in Maputsoe, a rapidly growing industrial township. Each FC would be staffed by a total of 12–14 persons, including a doctor, nurse clinician, and two double-qualified nurses. In Maseru, these personnel would be redeployed from the existing outpatient departments at QE II, which would be phased down and eventually closed.

To raise substantially the quality of service and increase the efficiency of expenditures at QE II, an integrated package (including infrastructure upgrading, equipment, training, technical assistance and organizational changes) would be implemented under the project. This subcomponent would be closely related to the establishment of urban filter clinics which would help to reduce the outpatient and maternity patient load at the central hospital. Physical and management improvements of the existing hospital would also be a significantly more affordable and cost-effective alternative to the construction of a new national referral hospital, which the government had earlier considered. A gradual phased approach to a new referral hospital would be studied further under the project.

Benefits Lesotho would benefit from increased efficiencies and some tangible savings in selected parts of the health service delivery system, as well as from higher cost recovery. Efficiency gains would emerge at facility level through management changes and adherence to unit cost targets, as well as from reforms of the drug system and goal of Ministry of Health staff as a part of improved manpower management. Savings would be realized through the utilization of lower cost peripheral health facilities and a reduction in referrals to QE II.

well identified slum areas of major cities including La Paz, Cochabamba and Santa Cruz in Bolivia, Calcutta, Delhi, and Madras in India, and Manila and Cebu in the Philippines; by building or upgrading primary care centres; and by training and deploying nurses and other paramedical staff and outreach workers, including community volunteers. The Philippines project goes beyond enhancing basic service provision for the poor, to developing the capacity of municipal governments to plan and manage health programmes for the urban poor. The first India project, described in greater detail in Box 8.2, also aims to strengthen the capacity of municipal Family Welfare Bureaus to deliver services, disseminate information and monitor progress.

By contrast, the Chile, Kenya and Tunisia projects concentrate mostly on measures to improve the efficiency of urban based hospitals. In Chile and Kenya, these hospitals are located entirely within the region of the capital city (Santiago and Nairobi, respectively), by far the largest metropolitan area in each country. A major underlying objective of these projects is to reallocate public spending for health from tertiary care to more cost-effective basic public health and clinical services for the poor.

This is to be done by increasing the utilization of lower level health centres and hospitals (as in Chile) and by raising cost recovery from the wealthy and insured who use tertiary care facilities (Tunisia). Both activities are being pursued in Kenya: the Kenyatta National Hospital is being upgraded, and at the same time a private practice wing with full cost user fees is being established at the hospital. The Tunisia project is described in greater detail in Box 8.3.

The other two projects, in Lesotho and Mozambique, are hybrids of the two approaches mentioned above. They attempt to improve access to basic health services for the urban poor by building neighbourhood health centres and training paramedics to staff these facilities; and they also involve rehabilitation and management reforms of the central hospitals in the capital cities of Maseru and Maputo, respectively. The Lesotho project is described in greater detail in Box 8.4.

COMPLEMENTARY WORLD BANK ACTIONS TO SUPPORT URBAN HEALTH GOALS

In addition to the rapid and significant growth in World Bank studies and projects for urban health outlined above, the Bank is also becoming increasingly involved in analysis and financial assistance in several other closely related sectors. These include urban development, water and sanitation, and the environment.

The 1992 *World Development Report* on the environment emphasized the negative impact on health of risk factors in the ambient environment but especially in the household environment: contaminated drinking water, inadequate sanitation and indoor air pollution from cooking fires (World Bank 1992b). The 1993 *World Development Report* built upon the previous Report, arguing for the first time that these risk factors in the household environment could be associated with nearly 30 per cent of the global burden of disease. The report suggested that feasible and affordable improvements in the household environment, in cities and in rural areas, could avert almost a quarter of this burden of disease, equivalent to reducing the number of infant deaths worldwide by about 2.5 million a year.

Both of these Reports were strongly influenced by the growing literature on the epidemiology of urban populations in the developing world. Much of this literature is well summarized in a study commissioned for the Urban Management and Environment component of the joint UNDP/World Bank/UNCHS Urban Management Programme. The study (Bradley et al 1992) made important strides in developing an environmental taxonomy that can be related to urban disease patterns and in summarizing the literature on intra-urban differentials in morbidity and mortality; on morbidity and mortality among vulnerable urban groups; and on the causal relationship between urban environmental conditions and morbidity and mortality.

Using these and other methodologies and building upon their policy recommendations, the Bank's lending for urban development and for water and sanitation have focused on urban based projects with mainly health objectives. In 1992, for example, two such urban development projects were launched: Lobito Benguela Urban Environmental Rehabilitation in Angola and Tianjin Urban Development and Environment in China. Concomitantly, the Bank approved four water and sanitation projects with explicit urban health goals: Water Sector Modernization in Brazil; Beijing Environment in China; Mombasa and Coastal Water Supply in Kenya; and Pujan and Taejon Sewerage in Korea.

PROSPECTS FOR THE FUTURE

Given the World Bank's strong commitment to poverty reduction and the momentum of ongoing studies, policy discussions and projects related to urban health, an increase in Bank involvement in the sector is virtually assured. Municipal health projects are already under preparation or ready for approval in a number of countries, including Argentina, Colombia and Venezuela.

As the World Bank enters increasingly into the arena of urban health, four key issues are likely to dominate the policy debate and practical design of programmes:

1. **Identifying the interventions that will have the greatest impact on the health of the urban poor**.

While these interventions will vary from country to country, depending on local epidemiology, the findings of the 1993 *World Development Report* suggest that a minimum package of basic services with high cost-effectiveness would have a major impact in reducing the current burden of disease in virtually all developing countries. This package includes health information, immunization, school health measures, prenatal and delivery care and family planning, treatments for sick children, and simple treatments for tuberculosis and sexually transmitted diseases. Countries need to begin using available information on cost-effectiveness of interventions in designing and implementing such packages of care. While many of the same health problems prevailing in rural communities will also affect the urban poor, the mortality and morbidity connected with violence, accidents and pollution will be greater in the urban setting. Intervention programmes will need to take these risk factors into account.

2. **Determining the appropriate role of the government and the private sector in delivering urban health services**.

While government financing of a basic package of public health and clinical care, especially for the poor, can be justified on both market failure and welfare grounds, the case for public financing of other health services is less compelling. User charges and unsubsidized insurance must be put in place, to ensure that the better off pay for these private services of lower cost-effectiveness. Similarly, even in situations where the government finances health care, this does not automatically mean that it should deliver it. On the contrary, the often dense urban networks of private providers – for profit modern physicians, traditional practitioners and NGOs – can do much to supply basic health services in the cities (for example, see the chapters by Atkinson, and Auer and Duncan). Government policies need to facilitate the actions of these private providers, not stifle them. This is one of the objectives of the World Bank urban health projects in India and the Philippines.

3. Targeting vital health services to the urban poor.

Targeting free or highly subsidized services can be achieved in many countries by concentrating these subsidies on facilities located in low income neighbourhoods. Untargeted supply of some services such as immunizations and tuberculosis therapy is inexpensive and has the advantage of maintaining political support from the better off. Universal subsidies for an enriched package of care also helps to enlist political support, as in Korea and Costa Rica, but will remain unaffordable in most developing countries. These twin issues of how much to target the poor and how exactly to do so – which instruments to use – will be central to the design of effective public policies for urban health.

4. Defining the respective responsibilities of urban local government and of central agencies such as health ministries in developing policies and managing health services in urban areas.

The evidence thus far suggests that this will depend on the capacity of municipal governments and the legal framework for delegating authority and financial resources. Where these are well developed, as in parts of Latin America, a central role for local government in planning and managing health services can lead to higher quality and greater efficiency, responsiveness and accountability. Where local capacity is weaker, as in much of Africa, a more gradual devolution will be required.

As the World Bank focuses more on urban health issues, it is establishing collaborations with a number of other aid agencies. For example, the Swiss government is actively involved in urban health activities in the Republic of Chad and Tanzania, and the United Kingdom's Overseas Development Administration is assisting in reforms of large hospitals in Lesotho, Zimbabwe, Zambia and other countries. The Inter American Development Bank is becoming increasingly active in urban health projects in Latin America. Effective collaboration between the Bank and these agencies is needed to improve the effectiveness of donor actions. Cofinancing of national programmes and of specific intervention projects, collaboration on urban health sector studies, joint donor reviews of implementation, and periodic meetings to discuss policies and reform activities in urban health are all important tools for improving donor performance.

It is clear that in recent years the World Bank and others have come to recognize the importance of urban health, and are beginning to appreciate the complexity of urban health policy issues. The commitment to do more and better exists. It now remains to translate that commitment into a series of increasingly effective policy recommendations and donor assisted programmes. Before the end of the current decade, we will be in a position to assess the effectiveness of urban health's contribution to overall development and poverty reduction.

REFERENCES

Barnum, H and Kutzin, J (1993) *Public Hospitals in Developing Countries: Resource Use, Cost, Financing* Johns Hopkins University Press, Baltimore

Bradley, D Cairncross, S Harpham, T and Stephens, C (1992) *A Review of Environmental Health Impacts in Developing Country Cities.* Urban Management Programme Paper 6, The World Bank, Washington DC

World Bank (1990a) *Brazil: The New Challenge of Adult Health* A World Bank Country Study, Washington DC

World Bank (1990b) *Poverty: The World Development Report 1990.* Oxford University Press, New York

World Bank (1991) *Kenya Hospital Rehabilitation Project* Staff Appraisal Report 9174-KE, Washington DC

World Bank (1992a) *China: Long-Term Issues and Options in the Health Transition* A World Bank Country Study, Washington DC

World Bank (1992b) *Development and the Environment: The World Development Report 1992* Oxford University Press, New York

World Bank (1992c) *Poverty Reduction Handbook* Washington DC

World Bank (1992d) *Zimbabwe: Financing Health Services* A World Bank Country Study, Washington DC

World Bank (1993) *Investing in Health: The World Development Report 1993* Oxford University Press, New York

9

The Evolution of UNICEF's Activities in Urban Health

R Padmini

INTRODUCTION

UNICEF's urban programme experience began in the late 1960s, and evolved by the 1970s into the Urban Basic Services (UBS) strategy, in more than 40 countries. During the last decade, UNICEF assistance to children and women in urban areas was expressed in various ways: support for national, centrally designed and sectoral services in urban areas such as Universal Child Immunization (UCI) and Oral Rehydration Therapy (ORT) drives; 'continued support for subnational, participatory and intersectoral Urban Basic Services programmes; greatly expanded efforts in favour of working and street children; country specific studies and assessments; and advocacy on macro-economic issues affecting the urban poor, as for example, "Adjustment With a Human Face". In the early 1990s, the Mayors' Initiative has called upon mayors to pursue the decade goals for their own cities by assessing the situation of their children, formulating subnational plans of action, and supporting community as well as sectoral initiatives' (UNICEF 1993).

In the 1980s, following the Alma Ata Primary Health Care (PHC) conference, UNICEF collaborated with WHO in sponsoring two interregional meetings on Urban Primary Health Care (see the chapter by Goldstein et al). These provided useful guidelines to countries as well as to international and national agencies interested in the health of the urban poor.

The UBS strategy has been the most systematic response from UNICEF to the problems of the urban poor, and their children, since the 1970s, and recognized by the UNICEF Executive Board as such (UNICEF 1986). 'The rationale for the urban focus of UNICEF has always been that the urban poor are among the most vulnerable, while at the same time they are highly resourceful and resilient and contribute significantly to urban and national development. Given some support, they can improve dramatically their situation and that of their children. Due to the peculiar urban conditions of density, cash economy, high proportion of female-headed households and lack of traditional community and extended family ties, appropriate mechanisms have to be devised for bringing development to the urban poor. Also, many poor families (urban as well as rural) have a number of child survival, development and protection problems. These various aspects of the problem faced by the urban poor called for convergent basic services, combined with strong community participation and family capacity building. Thus, a dual approach was adopted to bring direct services to the poor and to provide indirect services through training of government officials and service providers and advocating policy changes designed to help the urban poor' (UNICEF 1993, para 19).

Urban Basic Services is more than the sum of its parts. Its mutually reinforcing sectoral interventions are driven by objectives that ideally include:

- **community empowerment** through participation, organization, training and access to local government services;
- **universal coverage** of all target groups by sectoral services;
- **institutional linkages** through trained community volunteers and paraprofessionals which assure support for community services;
- **convergence of services** through intersectoral coordination of planning and service provision at the local level, and policy coordination at the national level;
- **advocacy** which succeeds in incorporating urban poor community needs into state policies and programmes;
- **use of low cost technologies** to ensure their continued use under local management;
- **capacity building** for communities, local government and national agencies to support services and community development in poor urban areas;
- **sustainability** that flows from the realization of the above objectives, especially empowerment, low cost technologies and capacity building;
- **institutionalization and 'going to scale'** through training, supporting community development and intersectoral coordination structures in local government, influencing national laws and policies toward the urban poor.

No single project can claim to have incorporated all these aspects successfully, but there are many examples of the synergy gained by several of them being combined in a good project.

URBAN BASIC SERVICES AND URBAN PHC

For UNICEF, UBS is almost a synonym for urban PHC, comprising as it does all the elements that make up PHC in the original sense expounded at Alma Ata. The cover of UNICEF's occasional 'Urban Examples' issue number 12, *Child Survival and Development and Urban Basic Services* brings out one way of looking at this relationship, as also with specific UNICEF concerns of the 1980s such as UCI and Child Survival and Development (CSD).

A triangle on its side (Figure 9.1) depicts UCI as the 'cutting edge' or the initial wedge of a programme which broadens out to include other components of the Child Survival and Development Revolution (CSDR) strategy, such as oral rehydration therapy and nutrition. CSD, in turn, can eventually fit into the supportive context of a community based primary health care system which includes water and sanitation as well as broader maternal and child health (MCH) elements. Finally, the PHC approach can be broadened even further to become a comprehensive, need based Basic Services programme including components as diverse and related as preschool education, income generating activities for women and female literacy.

In practice, UBS has always had a strong component of health, sanitation and hygiene, whether it starts from these aspects or moves on to them.

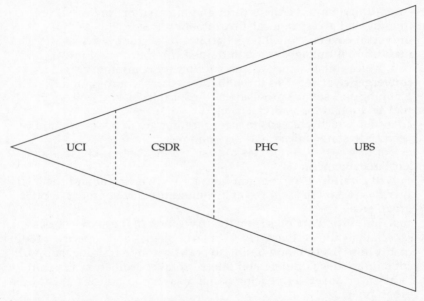

Figure 9.1 *From Child Survival to Urban Basic Services: the continuum of UNICEF's activities in urban health*

IMPLEMENTING URBAN SERVICES – EXAMPLES

Different patterns of linkages between sectoral goals and the UBS approach have emerged over time. In several countries, the UBS programme has embraced sectoral interventions and thus enabled a sharper focus on measurable goals. India's UBS programme provided the necessary social infrastructure and community involvement to facilitate other programmes. One example of this was the 1989 cholera epidemic in Delhi, when UBS volunteers supported by health workers managed to keep the death toll to one in 20,000 slum dwellers, while the city as a whole had 1300 deaths. Lima, Peru, had a similar experience in the 1991 cholera epidemic.

Moreover, in several countries, sectoral programmes were an 'entry point' for participatory development and service convergence. For example, in Tegucigalpa, Honduras, the *barrios marginales*, typically situated on the steep hillsides around the town, have to purchase water from private vendors, often at an estimated cost 34 times the official rate. The city water supply authorities built a community tank that would have been filled by them, and fed by gravity to public standpipes where the community would take over and sell the water at a rate far below the private vendors. The essence of this system was community (especially women's) participation, from the point of the request originating from the community to the administration of the water supply. These barrio residents have used the community organization so generated to move into other areas such as training health volunteers to run popular pharmacies and community child care services, and to demand services from the government. It is now planning ways to improve roads and sanitation.

UCI campaigns and oral rehydration therapy drives often reached their targets in urban areas, but only in a few cases served as entry points for the expansion and/or upgrading of urban health services, as, for example, in Turkey and in some towns in the Philippines (UNICEF 1992).

Multisectoral linkages are, however, not automatically established. UCI efforts in India and the Philippines did not use the UBS structures until the end of the 1980s, when special efforts had to be made in order to achieve the targets. These experiences have resulted in useful lessons regarding the need for community involvement in UCI or other goal achievement.

Still, examples abound, from the beginnings of UBS to the present day, of multisectoral projects. The Hyderabad Slum Improvement project in India, started in 1967, covered not only self-help housing improvements but provision of basic services, including health, women's economic activities and community organization. The Baldia project in Karachi, Pakistan constructed 6000 soakpits, and also developed 'home schools' for women, which led to economic activities.

In Peru, one of the UBS projects in Lima developed modules of services administered by community organizations, with volunteers trained as health agents, preschool animators and social communication facilitators. Early childhood development centres, health posts, popular kitchens and women's organizations were established.

A case study of ongoing UBS projects in three cities in Kenya – Nairobi, Mombasa and Kisumu – has noted the mutual support of the community health organization and the formal health system, within a multisectoral framework. While community health workers have been trained to distribute contraceptives and drugs to prevent diseases such as malaria, outreach clinics established through the programme have significantly raised levels of immunization and lowered the infant mortality rate. Other project activities include nutritional rehabilitation of severely malnourished children, nutrition education for expectant and lactating women, early childhood education centres, ventilated improved pit latrines, and water kiosks or piped water.

Women's groups have been highly instrumental in the successes of UBS. They often function as health and early child care volunteers. Their special concerns include monitoring of immunization, prenatal care, providing health education and ORT, and maintaining the local water supply. In slums in Turkey, their collective action in demanding better garbage collection was successful. In Indonesia, block grants have been used for PHC and nonformal education for mothers in urban slum areas.

The policy review of 1993 noted that 'successful UBS projects have expanded in Indonesia and the Philippines and have attracted funds' (in Hyderabad, India, 13 times the initial amount provided by UNICEF and the Government). They have also spawned other projects and have been instrumental in national acceptance of the overall concept. Since the 1970s, UBS in India has spread from three initial towns to 168 towns and has been incorporated in the national development plan. The Philippines urban pro-poor programme is also patterned on the UBS approach. Similar expansions are found in Colombia, Ethiopia and Central America.

Constraints to Urban Basic Services

- In many cases, the need to build community confidence has led UBS programmes to focus on the process of community development rather than on the impact on children and women.
- The UBS approach takes time for major impacts to be felt.
- UBS works primarily at the community level, and sometimes does not link up with national sectoral programmes. On the other hand, such national programmes do not easily connect with community based programmes. Working on a multisectoral programme with multiple partners in the government and outside is inherently difficult. Effecting such linkages remains a key challenge.
- Though community based baseline surveys have been invaluable for community empowerment and action, monitoring and evaluation have consisted mainly of anecdotal evidence of the gains and shortcomings of projects, and of the approach itself. More attention to costs, including community contributions is needed.
- Most UBS projects are initially small in size and few have gone to scale with speed. Yet this is a process that has to be nurtured carefully as there are pitfalls in rapid expansion. The very features (community empowerment, convergence and locally managed approaches) that make UBS efficacious may suffer when going to scale.

UNICEF'S CURRENT URBAN POLICY

The key features of the UNICEF revised urban policy that was approved by its Board in 1993 are:

1. the poor urban child should be a key concern in all sectoral programmes; and
2. a revitalized UBS strategy should be pursued, building on its successes and seizing new opportunities for expansion.

'Both principles should be derived from a country's National Plan of Action (NPA), with the sectoral programmes striving to reach all urban children, while the UBS strategy focuses specifically on the poor through innovative, viable approaches and supports links between community and provider.'

Thus the two-pronged urban strategy that is now the UNICEF policy seeks to maximize the opportunities for both building upon the experiences of UBS and bringing the sectoral interventions to hitherto unreached or poorly served urban areas and populations, while utilizing the lessons learnt through UBS approaches. In the former case, the idea is that UNICEF will continue to support national and international efforts to plan and implement community based multisectoral programmes in the poorer urban areas. In the latter case, UNICEF will work with appropriate national ministries and other sectoral institutions to strive to effectively reach *all* urban children *as needed*. The UBS type of programmes cover only a fraction of the children of the urban poor and even if expanded rapidly, could not cover all of them within this decade. Hence the sectoral interventions could aim at such blanket coverage.

The World Summit plan of action for children had envisaged national, sectoral and subnational plans of action based upon the global plan, but adapted to the differing situations. UNICEF's new urban policy envisages that UNICEF should strive for this focus through support to NPAs and sectoral plans in order to examine the country's urban problems and assess the impact of policies and programmes on urban children, with special reference to those in low income areas. Given that urban social services are generally under the authority of the municipality, though at the same time the private sector and NGOs are key actors, all three groups need to cooperate to ensure the success of both routine services and special campaigns.

Municipal plans of action, based upon each country's NPA, are proposed to be prepared with the collaboration of these various actors and community groups. The Mayor's Initiative is seen as a special opportunity to do so.

In the health area, there is a need to assess local patterns of disease, indicators of morbidity and mortality, and data regarding occupation, shelter and environment, as each type of urban area, and even each city, may be different. 'The role of such providers as national government, municipal government, health insurers, formal sector and workers' benefit schemes, private practitioners, informal providers and existing community based health systems have to be taken into account. As urban health problems are closely tied to the environment, a multisectoral approach, coordinated at the municipal level, needs to be adopted' (UNICEF 1993).

Since natural increase has increasingly become the major contributor to urban growth in the past decade, support to government and United Nations Population Fund programmes has been cited as necessary. The 'baby-friendly' hospital initiative which seeks to have all hospitals and health centres practise the ten steps to successful breastfeeding needs to be supplemented by community and institutional support to aid urban mothers, especially working mothers, by providing crèche and day care services, paid postnatal leave and flexible working hours.

The policy paper similarly envisages that other sectors, such as education, social welfare, and water and sanitation, need a deliberate assessment and refocusing in the urban areas, especially the poorer urban areas, in order that the year 2000 goals for children can be achieved. 'Addressing the inequities in the provision of urban social services will necessitate the following four types of action which target the poor:

1. restructuring sector resources in favour of low cost technologies and approaches;
2. advocacy and support for institutional capacity building, community participation/management and promotion of such innovative approaches as linkage with income-generating activities;
3. lifting subsidies to the better off to facilitate subsidization of services to the poor and using innovative, soft recyclable loans to accelerate coverage of the unserved; and
4. promotion and support of intra- and interregional exchange of innovative ideas and approaches, as well as technical cooperation among developing countries.

'Sectoral programmes and their staff should be oriented to deal with communities and local government. Close interaction between these programmes and UBS and other community based programmes should be encouraged; in addition, specific training and exchange of experience must be carried out. Sectoral components of UNICEF country programmes need to include a specific urban focus so as to support the thrust of the sectoral and subnational NPAs' (UNICEF 1993).

A REVITALIZED URBAN BASIC SERVICES STRATEGY

The need to revitalize the UBS strategy is to enable a proven approach to go to scale, have greater impact upon the well being of children and women, and tie in with other forces so as to help tackle some of the root problems of the urban poor. It consists 'of four key thrusts within the framework of the NPA and the country programme approach:

1. promotion of the decade goals for children while joining other partners in poverty reduction (especially to aid working mothers);
2. application of the Agenda-21 concept of Primary Environmental Care (PEC) in low income urban areas;
3. support to both rehabilitative and preventive approaches for children in especially difficult circumstances; and
4. advocacy, technical support and applied research for 'urban development with a human face'.

'In order to go to scale in the achievement of these goals, efforts will include the development of viable national urban policies; capacity building for local level management of sustainable urban development; and improved monitoring and impact analysis with attention to the costs of UBS to both service providers and to households' (UNICEF 1993).

Promotion of children's goals and partnerships for poverty alleviation

The first of the four key thrusts in the revitalized UBS strategy, ie, achievement of the decade goals for children and partnerships for poverty alleviation, is in fact an extension of the UBS approach already in place in several countries. The poor are doubly affected in a cash economy – by the need to pay cash for every service and by the opportunity costs of the time needed to utilize the service. Hence the achievement of the decade goals for children can have a dual benefit for the urban poor – by improving their children's survival, development and protection, while at the same time reducing the economic burden of children's illnesses and helping to alleviate poverty. If these actions are based upon community participation and capacity building, the benefits will be sustained. These tasks will need the support of many agencies, and UNICEF will work with others both to attain the decade goals and to launch a broadbased attack on poverty.

In the health area, a preventive approach that obviates the need for the poor to devote insufferable amounts of time or cash must be promoted. This has been found in practice to need a combination of a community based system that uses simply trained workers who are either part time and voluntary or full time and paid by some form of charge to the community, and access to the first line of referral of the formal health structure. Links between the community workers and the urban health system must be carefully worked out.

The 'baby-friendly' hospital initiative is by itself not sufficient to ensure the infant's nutritional advancement. Most low income urban mothers need to get back to work almost immediately after childbirth, and innovative locally devised and managed child care systems are needed to see that she can continue to exclusively breastfeed for at least four months. After that age, too, care of the young child is a prime concern as options often used by low income urban mothers are to leave the child with an older sibling, an aged relative or even alone. Community based child care in UBS areas has been promoted and found to be successful in promoting child health and development, apart from helping the mother to do her work outside the home. A specific urban nutritional issue is the promotion and easy availability of appropriate low cost weaning foods. Careful use of mass media, *Facts for Life* and other social communication tools geared to urban life are also needed, in support of community based nutritional surveillance and growth promotion.

Primary Environmental Care

The Primary Environmental Care (PEC) concept, that has evolved in relation to the environmental concerns in the past several years, and UBS are mutually reinforcing concepts. PEC focuses on fulfillment of basic needs, thus supporting efforts to achieve the decade goals, but adding a more explicit concern for environmental improvements and management. Its emphasis on community empowerment is also congruent with UBS principles. An example of the PEC approach is in looking at preventive health care in dense, low income urban areas. Such an approach would not only support the use of low cost, locally managed technologies in the provision of safe water supply and disposal of solid and liquid waste, but add a special emphasis on environmentally sustainable practices (that would in fact lead to both health benefits and savings) (Environment & Urbanization 1992). For example, some urban community groups have been hygienically recycling inorganic waste and composting organic garbage, using hand carts or animal-driven ones; this has provided employment, and the compost has been used in urban agriculture (UNICEF 1993).

Another area of urban concern is air pollution. While some types of urban air pollution can be tackled only by city-wide systems, alternative fuels, improved stoves and planting of trees on a small scale can be promoted, creating both health and economic benefits.

Children in Especially Difficult Circumstances and 'Urban Development with a Human Face'

In this paper, it is only possible and necessary to touch upon the other two 'key thrusts' of the revitalized UBS strategy: Children in Especially Difficult Circumstances (CEDC) and 'Urban Development with a Human Face'. Rehabilitative approaches for CEDC focus on community and street based action to support and rehabilitate them. As for prevention, alternative educational, as well as recreational, schemes are proposed to be stressed through UBS. However, the structural causes of poverty and conflict need wider onslaughts, and UBS can only try to help in that much bigger effort through its advocacy.

UNICEF vigorously advocated 'Adjustment with a Human Face' in the 1980s, calling for modifying structural adjustment measures by the provision of safety nets for the poor. This approach has evolved in the 1990s into advocacy and policy support for 'Development with a Human Face', which clearly must include urban development. UNICEF will, along with other partners concerned with human development and poverty reduction, play an advocacy and technical support role in the development of viable national urban policies. Such a focus on the urban poor must be set in the context of a balanced urban and rural strategy, in the interests of comprehensive national development.

SOME ONGOING INITIATIVES

As a followup to the World Summit for Children in 1990, many countries have prepared their National Plans of Action. While these vary a great deal, they are mostly general statements of intent, and are expected to be followed up by more specific sectoral and subnational plans of action. In fact, some countries have already taken steps to prepare these. There is a plan of action for Mexico City; draft plans of action exist for four Bangladesh urban centres. These typically address health, nutrition and water and sanitation problems, as well as other sectors such as education and sometimes CEDC. Another type of reference to urban concerns is in a country's NPA itself. For example, in the Indian NPA, there are several references to the special needs of urban slum areas.

Running parallel to this process of preparation of subnational and specifically municipal plans of action, has been the Mayors' Initiative. Inspired by the Convention on the Rights of the Child, several Italian mayors pledged in 1990 to become 'Defenders of Children'. This idea was taken up by two international colloquia held in Dakar, Senegal in January 1992 and in Mexico City in July 1993, respectively (UNICEF 1993). These commitments by the municipal leadership need to be followed up by specific city plans of action that are implemented and monitored. UNICEF country offices will work with the mayors concerned on these steps. Further, the participants of the two colloquia are called upon to hold national and regional meetings and to involve other mayors in this initiative.

While the Mayors' Initiative declarations and plans of action cover the various goals derived from the World Summit of 1990, the Mexico statement has a sharper focus on the mid-decade or intermediate goals. Most of these goals are in the health field, especially with reference to disease control or eradication. The nutrition and water and sanitation goals are obviously closely linked to health improvements. These intermediate goals have been endorsed by the UNICEF-WHO Joint Committee on Health Policy in 1993. This meeting also emphasized the need to have 'special programmes for populations at risk or uncovered; programmes for urban slums.

One of the followup actions on the intermediate goals is to hold regional meetings of country and regional staff of the two organizations including the WHO Representatives and UNICEF Urban and Health Programme Officers at the country level to discuss joint action plans to support countries in the achievement of the decade goals and the mid-decade goals in urban areas.

UNICEF has been following the Healthy Cities initiative supported by WHO (see the chapter by Goldstein et al) with interest over the years, and with a number of developing countries taking up this idea, could work on it with WHO in many countries. Here it is worth noting the broad congruence of the Healthy Cities approach with that of UBS.

OPERATIONAL STEPS TOWARDS GOAL ACHIEVEMENT/SUSTAINABILITY IN URBAN AREAS

Apart from the operational steps towards achievement and sustainability of the decade and mid-decade goals in urban areas noted in the previous sections, UNICEF has also been involved in discussion with other partners such as UNDP, the World Bank and UNCHS regarding collaboration on reaching the goals for children. UNFPA and WFP who are also active in the urban areas, as well as several bilateral governmental and Non-governmental agencies need also to be involved in such partnership. On the national side, followup is needed on the NPAs, the sectoral NPAs and the city plans of action (especially if the mayor has attended one of the two Mayors' Initiative colloquia, or any regional or national one).

UNICEF country offices are preparing workplans to outline how they will support national efforts to achieve the goals. The urban staff in

UNICEF at headquarters, as well as at the field level, will be paying special attention to strategies and activities aimed at reaching the urban population, particularly the urban poor. The field offices will also support as appropriate, national or regional mayors' meetings to spread the idea of the Mayors' Initiative. Many country programmes assisted by UNICEF have expanded UBS or initiated them. It will be especially important to see that these incorporate the new policy guidelines for urban programmes.

These tasks are being seen as a global collaborative effort not simply the tasks of the small advisory group at UNICEF Headquarters or even of the entire UNICEF staff. The only hope for rapid expansion of the UBS approach is for all agencies who are convinced by it to adopt it as their own, improve upon it and spread it far and wide.

REFERENCES

Environment & Urbanization (1992) Sustainable Cities: meeting needs, reducing resource use and recycling, re-use and reclamation, vol 4, no 2, October

UNICEF (1993) *Programmes for the Urban Poor* Report no E/ICEF/1993/L.9 UNICEF, New York

UNICEF (1986) *Urban Basic Services: Reaching Children and Women of the Urban Poor* Report by the Executive Director, UNICEF, Occasional Papers Series no 3 UNICEF, New York

UNICEF (1992) *The Antalya Gecekondu Project: A Progress, Crises and Prospects Report* UNICEF, Turkey, June; Pacifico (Pax) F Maghacot, Jr *A Case Study of the UNICEF-Assisted Urban Basic Services Programme in the Philippines* Manila, Philippines, October

UNICEF (1992) Mayors for Children, International Colloquium of Mayors, Dakar, Senegal, 8–9 January 1992; Mayors Defenders of Children, Mexico City, 5–7 July 1993

10

USAID's Experience in Urban Health and Directions for the Future

Holly Fluty and Jennifer Lissfelt*

INTRODUCTION

In this chapter, we outline the US Agency for International Development's (USAID) support for urban health activities, lessons learned from past and ongoing urban health efforts, and likely future efforts and priorities for the Agency in the urban health area. We attempt to show the evolution of this topic within the Agency by considering specifically the activities of the Agency's Office of Health. Although other USAID Washington Offices, such as Population and Housing and Urban Programmes, also have experience in urban health-related efforts, their activities are largely separate from the Office of Health and Nutrition and will not be examined in this chapter.

OVERVIEW OF US GOVERNMENT FOREIGN ASSISTANCE

The United States Agency for International Development was created by Congress in 1961 under the Foreign Assistance Act (FAA) as a semi-autonomous agency of the US Department of State to coordinate and manage all foreign economic assistance activities, with a focus on helping the rural poor. The Agency was established within the Department of State, and is headed by an Administrator who, as a Presidential Appointee, reports to the President and on issues of foreign policy and overall coordination reports to the Secretary of State.

In devising its development activities, USAID is faced with three major difficulties:

1. overall foreign policy considerations and the political nature of

---

* The ideas and opinions expressed in this chapter are those of the authors and should not be attributed to the US Agency for International Development.

assistance, with consequent apportionment of foreign assistance
funding;
2. the long, multiyear planning process which can make programmes
   obsolete or inflexible to changing events; and
3. the reality of annual budget appropriations from Congress which
   often fall short of resources needed to accomplish all that has been
   proposed.

Foreign policy and USAID'S mandate

The Foreign Assistance Act as it is currently written contains many
different objectives for United States economic assistance (over 30).
Members of Congress and others have noted that with so many objectives
it is difficult to have a clear direction or goal, and to implement plans
effectively. Over the 30 years of its existence, USAID's goals and objectives
have grown substantially – and, for the most part, rather than omitting
certain objectives, as new ones developed they have merely been added to
pre-exisiting objectives. This has hindered USAID's ability to focus its
efforts and to meet its many mandates from Congress and interest groups.

USAID funds are apportioned according to national interests and
foreign policy objectives. Therefore, in the post Cold War era, while the
biggest aid recipients are still Israel and Egypt, assistance is rising
dramatically for Russia and the New Independent States of the former
Soviet Union; needs are also emerging for southern Africa and West
Bank/Gaza activities. It has been said that '[Foreign assistance] is now
largely military and security, directed to countries which can be served
by other mechanisms of US cooperation, and is not directed to where
most of the people are in need' (Berg 1989 p33).

There have been three major periods of US foreign assistance as the
aid programme changed with American domestic concerns and
international realities: 1948–1952 (Marshall Plan years – $35 billion per
year), 1953–1973 (stable $22 billion per year), 1976–present (considerable
fluctuation, but average of $15 billion per year). Despite US public and
congressional concerns over levels of foreign aid spending, foreign aid
was only 3 per cent of GNP in 1949, slightly more than 1 per cent during
the 1950s, and has fallen every year since 1965 to its current level of
approximately 0.25 per cent (Hamilton 1989 p28). The US is in last place
among the OECD nations in its foreign aid–GNP ratio.

Planning process

Foreign economic assistance through USAID undergoes an intensive
planning process years in advance of programme implementation.
USAID has planning cycles of two to three years for country development
strategies which results in many activities becoming obsolete or requiring
modification as events change. USAID's planning process also involves
many stakeholders, including the US Congress through its oversight of
specified funding for special interest areas and for designated countries.
The focus on these emphasis areas limits the flexibility of USAID in
geographic scope, programmes and funding levels.

Budget realities

USAID makes an annual presentation to Congress to request funds for the following fiscal year. Of the three branches of the US Government, only Congress can authorize funds, with the Executive Branch proposing annual budgets. USAID must respond to congressional interests as well as to the objectives of the current administration through the Department of State. Such a response results in USAID changing many of its policies and directions with every administration – and fighting for funding in an increasingly budget-conscious, anti foreign aid atmosphere. Hence, the reality is that USAID must work within political and budget considerations, and cannot develop its programmes or provide aid to countries solely on the basis of development measures or indicators.

USAID provides support primarily through a multifaceted structure comprised of USAID Washington, country missions and regional offices. The Agency's emphasis is on the field offices, ie missions, which have semi-autonomous country level decision making responsibility. USAID Washington provides policy and technical support, but in most cases does not initiate country activities without approval of the missions involved. USAID policy is established by the Programme and Policy Coordination Bureau; missions, regional and central bureaus cannot write policy for the Agency.

USAID Washington is divided into geographic regional bureaus and central bureaus including the Global Programmes, Field Support and Research Bureau to support technical activities of USAID around the world. Both the Office of Health and Nutrition and the Office of Population are involved in issues related to urban health and have some overlap in their activities – all fall under the Global Bureau.

Missions develop and implement programmes with host country governments and institutions, providing USAID with one of its greatest strengths as well as a comparative advantage since no other donor has such a staff presence in so many countries. USAID can, through its missions, have its finger on the pulse of local conditions and stay abreast of issues by communicating regularly with local experts and representatives. USAID's structure provides great possibilities for cooperation, concerted effort and broad presence, but it can also lead to conflict and division over USAID priorities and strategies to accomplish them.

USAID'S HEALTH PROGRAMMES

Under the Foreign Assistance Act of 1961, USAID's health mandate was to work with governments and incorporate health activities into other economic development activities. Such a directive recognized that healthy people can be more productive and greater productivity is a critical part of economic development.

Section 104(c)(1) of the 1961 FAA authorizes USAID's health activities, stating that:

> *Assistance under this subsection shall be used primarily for basic integrated health services, safe water and sanitation, disease prevention and control, and related health planning and research. The assistance shall emphasize self-sustaining community based health programmes by means such as training of health auxiliaries and other appropriate personnel, support for the establishment and evaluation of projects that can be replicated on a broader scale, measures to improve management of health programmes, and other services and suppliers to support health and disease prevention programmes.*

Despite a growing awareness of the urban poor in the 1980s and the emergence of proliferating urban slums and urban health problems as a critical issue, USAID's policies have continued to focus on rural initiatives. USAID's 1982 Health Assistance Policy Paper, which remains the policy in use today, states that 'the urban oriented, hospital based system has not proven an effective vehicle for improving general health conditions.' (p4) Thus the focus was, and is, on steering away from the cities towards basic health improvements for the harder to reach rural populations. The urban poor have not been given any visibility at the Agency's policy level; there has been little acknowledgement that the urban poor are as much or more high risk and low access as the rural poor.

USAID's Washington Office of Health and Nutrition and country based bilateral programmes (in accordance with specific country settings) focus their efforts on the following priority areas:

• child survival;
• maternal and reproductive health;
• HIV/AIDS;
• environmental health;
• health care system support and policy; and
• nutrition.

USAID intends to maintain its focus on 'broad delivery of proven interventions to improve child health but will give increased attention to the institutions, policy reform and financial base needed to sustain these programmes over the long term.' (USAID 1982, p8) However, this focus does not acknowledge segments of populations that have been missed by successful USAID activities, and that many problems of access and availability still have not been solved. Of growing recognition is that broad delivery will not be enough: once there is a sufficient quantity of services, the Agency needs to examine their quality and use by underserved and high risk groups – such as the urban poor.

USAID'S DEVELOPMENT STRATEGIES OVER TIME

Early years

Throughout the 1960s development assistance focused on macro-economic growth policies, gap models, infrastructure projects, institution building, green revolution technologies, agriculture and food for peace, and eradication of malaria and smallpox and other diseases. In these years, USAID's priorities in the health area were eradication and control of epidemic and endemic diseases (measles, smallpox, malaria, cholera), studying major causes of infant and child mortality, eliminating malnutrition, reducing population growth, developing training and research facilities, and developing water and sewage systems to reduce disease incidence from pollution.

USAID played an active role in the substantial collaboration among various international organizations in the worldwide malaria eradication programme, which was initiated in 1955. In the 1960s population programmes became very active and a major component of USAID's programme. A separate Population Office was created, and funds were earmarked for population initiatives. In 1962, USAID's Office of Housing and Urban Programmes was created. Since the 1960s, one of the focus areas of USAID's health programme has been water and sanitation and communicable disease research. This focus continues in the 1990s.

New directions

In the late 1960s and early 1970s, USAID began to change. The war in Vietnam brought a politicization of the Agency, and various country programmes indicated the need for changes in overall strategies. For example, it was becoming clear that traditional reliance on 'trickle-down' development and the belief that positive effects of growth would benefit the entire population were misguided. Many USAID officials began to recognize that the poor were often not benefiting from economic growth in their societies. It was believed that to help the poor, what was needed was to provide them with public services and to empower them. Integrated rural development grew out of this theory: reach inaccessible people, empower them, and use local labour. It was also in this time period that primary health care (PHC) became an important strategy of the Agency.

In 1971, USAID's PHC strategy began, with the goal of creating the broadest possible health benefits for the largest possible number of people in developing countries. The strategy focused on preventive health care and creation of feasible, sustainable health technologies. This new emphasis was further encouraged by the FAA of 1973 (termed the 'New Directions') which, in addition to other changes in USAID's mandate and regulations, emphasized basic human needs focusing on the rural poor. USAID's health activities began to be developed with more affordability, accessibility and equity in mind. At this time, there was a general reorientation within the development community away from high technology and building hospitals toward PHC in rural areas. Many activities took place under this general theme, including the Alma Ata conference and WHO's 'Health for All by the Year 2000' programme.

A significant health event in the 1970s was the eradication of smallpox around the world in 1977. The US played a major role in this effort through the US Centers for Disease Control and the success of the smallpox eradication programme generated interest in other health problems, including the possibility of eradicating other diseases.

The rural bias

USAID development efforts have for many years been dominated by rural oriented agriculturalists; USAID's, and indeed most of the development community's, health focus has long been on rural health. Urban dwellers have been perceived to be elites or middle class with better access to advanced health care and other services. In addition to proximity to facilities and services, urban dwellers have been viewed as privileged in that they have enjoyed benefits of infrastructure improvements, schools, tertiary care facilities and other advancements in living standards.

The continued emphasis in USAID was on moving efforts out of the cities to the countryside, to reach those not benefiting from the growth of cities and economies. It was also thought that this would take care of urbanization problems – helping the people in the countryside might keep them from migrating to urban areas.

There has been a fear that without a concerted effort to reach rural citizens, urban dwellers would – for reasons of access, financial ability and sophistication – reap all the rewards of development initiatives, and rural activities such as agriculture would continue to be taxed to subsidize urban infrastructure. Thus efforts were made by USAID to *counter the urban bias* – to 'level the playing field' for the rural people. There were increasing calls for rural infrastructure developments and equitable land distribution to bring growth, lower income inequality and decrease poverty. Countries such as Taiwan and Korea, with their rapid rural industrialization and high income equality, showed strong evidence in support of this approach.

1980s to the present

In the 1980s, there were major shifts in USAID activities in the development arena. The 1979 debt crisis brought a shift to the right in world power, election of more conservative leaders (eg, Reagan, Thatcher, Kohl), and less liberal thinking among developed country policy makers. In the early 1980s, the global recession decreased the availability of funds from governments to provide social services. One of the most significant outcomes of these events was recognition of the private sector as an important player – and provider of services – in development.

About this time, USAID's PHC strategy began to be less of a focus. In 1982, USAID policy shifted substantially when the Agency's Health Policy Paper stated that biomedical research on developing country diseases was a new emphasis. Although USAID had done some work in medical research, this new policy led to a substantial increase in research support that is still in evidence today. USAID's biomedical research work has moved beyond malaria vaccine to include measles and rotovirus vaccine research, diarrhoeal disease research and research into other diseases prevalent in countries where the Agency worked. Other areas under the new health policy included an official orientation away from the cities toward the rural areas, and improved effectiveness and self-financing of health programmes. This was a shift from the earlier focus on health commodities and infrastructure, and involved a new emphasis on private sector approaches. Health care financing became a focus area for USAID.

Also in the 1980s, with its lower ranking among international development donors, USAID became more aware of other donors' activities (Bissell 1989) and areas for potential collaboration. Such a recognition created a greater emphasis on policy dialogue and donor coordination. Although the United States was no longer the leader in the health field, its assistance in this sector traditionally has been grant and not loan funds, thus maintaining a significant voice despite being overtaken by other donors.

In the 1980s, both HIV/AIDS activities and the Child Survival Programme were initiated. Since 1985, USAID has devoted more than $1.5 billion dollars to child survival in more than 60 countries.

During the 1980s, as is the case today, the rural bias in USAID economic development programmes prevailed. Many current USAID staff were hired in the 1970s, when development policy had a rural orientation, and they therefore have an intrinsic rural focus. However, the issue of the urban poor and their health began to surface and become increasingly evident as an emerging area for development work. In 1988, Congress asked USAID to conduct a study to assess the potentially adverse effects of urbanization on development, and the ability of USAID and other donors' programmes to address these negative effects. This request showed a growing recognition of the changing demographics and epidemiology in the Third World, and of the fact that urbanization was accelerating and diseases were spreading more rapidly in high-density areas.

HOW HAS URBAN HEALTH EVOLVED AS A TOPIC FOR USAID?

The topic of urban health is a relatively new one for USAID and one that is beginning to develop, without any clear direction or official policy. USAID recognizes the needs of the urban poor and has made statements to this effect in publications such as the 1992 Child Survival Report to Congress: 'As the proportion and number of urban poor increase in coming years, new ways must be found to address their health and nutritional needs' (USAID 1992 p30). However, USAID does not have a policy on urban health, and many Agency officials are not yet familiar with the demographics and the implications of this issue for the future.

Within USAID, the interest in urban health issues and health care for the urban poor lies mainly with officers who have studied the topic, attended conferences, and examined the implications of this crisis for the future of Agency programmes. The issue has emerged repeatedly over the years, in the form of isolated efforts within USAID projects or stand-alone bilateral programmes, but as yet no cohesive Agency strategy has been devised to address it.

USAID's visible interest in the topic of health of the urban poor began in 1986, as an outgrowth of a USAID-funded conference developed by the National Council for International Health (NCIH). This conference can be considered an important milestone in the development of USAID's interest in urban health. The topic was seen as an emerging area, and one in which USAID could play a role. The conference was specifically geared toward private voluntary organizations (PVOs) working in urban health, and was entitled 'Health of the Urban Poor in Developing Countries: A Challenge to Private Voluntary Organizations.' At this conference, the USAID perspective was presented as being interested in the urban poor, given the realities of inefficient governments and poorly run public health systems not providing services to this population subset, as well as inappropriate health resource allocation and financing that focused more on high technology and curative care rather than effective public health measures for the populations most in need.

The USAID Washington Office of Health not only sponsored the conference but followed up by bringing attention to the issue through ongoing USAID health projects. The discussions resulted in urban health efforts that grew naturally out of projects with potential expertise in this area such as a project that focused on water and sanitation issues. Because USAID projects are designed with some flexibility to adapt efforts to current needs, these projects were able to have new activities that focused on the urban poor.

In 1991, USAID Washington held three conferences on the topic of urban health: 'Health in the Urban Setting' in Washington in March; 'Urban Health: Sharpening the Focus' in Washington in June; and 'AID Workshop on Urban Health and Environment in Africa' in Nairobi in December. Organized by the Office of Health, these three events heightened the realization of the critical urban health issues to be faced and the importance of future efforts in this area.

Due largely to diminishing staff and funding, USAID has not held any significant events and has designed few cohesive activities in urban health since these three conferences. However, USAID health projects and grants have continued to address problems of urbanization in conjunction with their other activities; and new projects have been designed with urban health and 'reaching high risk populations' elements built into them.

EXAMPLES OF USAID'S EFFORTS TO DATE

It is interesting to note that most USAID projects and programmes operate in capital cities and secondary cities and include urban elements, without many staff believing that they are involved in 'urban health' work *per se*. The Agency's approach to date has been relatively *ad hoc*, building urban efforts into projects as needs warranted or interest was recognized. However, USAID has found that 'where child survival programmes have addressed urban health issues, the rewards have been substantial' (USAID 1992 p29).

USAID has had several projects with urban health elements, including both centrally funded and bilateral projects. Some of these have been more successful than others. Key efforts, and lessons learned from a selection of the activities, are described below.

Bilateral efforts

Bangladesh Urban Volunteer Programme (1986–1991). This project was implemented through a grant to the International Centre for Diarrhoeal Disease Research, Bangladesh (ICDDR, B) to train female urban health volunteers (UVs) to provide child survival services to infants and children in the Dhaka slums. The project initially focused on controlling diarrhoeal diseases through ORS and health education, then expanded to include nutrition, immunization, family planning and an urban surveillance system. Approximately 2000 women from the slum areas (who had been recommended as good candidates for community service) were trained at ICDDR, B. The UVs were trained to provide services door-to-door. Although urban areas had been behind rural areas in immunization rates in 1988, by 1991 urban areas had higher rates than the rest of the country.

> *Lessons learned:* 1. *Need for low cost, community based solutions to assure sustainability of health interventions in urban poor communities. 2. Need to specifically target urban poor women for preventive health strategies. 3. Urban poor women are effective outreach workers and community motivators to reach other urban poor women. 4. Urban poor women are highly motivated, untapped resources with high development potential. 5. Urban health strategies need to be multifocal, involving community development, personal empowerment and infrastructure development. 6. Empowerment is gained through implementation of realistic household level interventions. 7. Health facility and water and sanitation infrastructure development combined with household level interventions through empowered populations are necessary to effect and maintain improvement in health status of urban poor.*

Bangladesh Family Planning and Health Services In the 1980s, Bangladesh, like many other countries, decided to strive for Universal Childhood Immunization, which would increase vaccination levels to 80 per cent for children under one year of age by 1990. However, Bangladesh began with one of the lowest coverage rates in the world: 2 per cent. The MOH, with donor support, implemented a plan which included phased activities in rural upazilas, regular visits by immunization workers, training of health workers and a social marketing campaign. However, urban children had been forgotten in the initial planning. After the first year, the MOH realized this and invited USAID to lead donor participation in the urban effort. USAID's major goal was to reaffirm the national policy and strategy, but make adjustments for the specific EPI needs of the country's 88 urban areas. Results were striking. In less than one year, urban EPI coverage in the phased areas, which had been severely lagging behind rural rates, caught up and then surpassed those in the identified upazilas. The national effort has been successful on a scale never before witnessed in Bangladesh. By 1990, Bangladesh did indeed advance coverage to 80 per cent.

Lessons learned: 1. *National EPI planners cannot assume that they will routinely effectively cover urban dwellers. This is the case in Bangladesh, where the four largest cities are specifically designated to take care of their own health needs without MOH intervention. 2. There is a need to address responsibilities between two concerned ministries: the MOH, which has national responsibility for health care in the country, and the technical expertise to provide services; and the Ministry of Local Government, which is the umbrella ministry for municipalities. As EPI grew in urban Bangladesh, it became clear that, while the MOH may have the technical knowledge and supplies to implement EPI, the cities themselves have the greater potential to ensure sustainable EPI and provide long term EPI staff, because they understand how their own cities function. This is a new role for many cities, and one which requires significant support by both ministries and individual cities. 3. Donors have little experience supporting municipal social service programmes. Although there is a wealth of experience in working with national level ministries, no donor had ever worked at such a scale to assist municipal governments.*

Egypt: Urban Health Delivery Systems (UHDS) This Cairo project, which ran from 1979 to 1988, was developed to demonstrate ways to improve health service accessibility and effectiveness, and to be replicable in other urban areas. The project concentrated on Helwan, South and West Cairo districts. The project's assumption was that if higher quality, more effective services were available locally, the people would use them more, and their health would improve. Project accomplishments included construction and renovation of all designated facilities in urban areas; and improved patient care, records and management systems in these facilities. Although the project focused on construction, rather than on delivery of services or training, the facilities have seen increased usage within target areas as a result of the project. Statistics point to higher life expectancy, reduced fertility and decreased infant mortality in the poor urban areas targeted by the project over a ten year period. The project made efforts to develop training, community participation, local delivery of health services, and health infrastructure improvements in Cairo and Alexandria. The project targeted three million people, most of whom were children under five and women of reproductive age.

Lessons learned: 1. *Given the complexity of the urban setting, the project design was too complicated and unrealistic. 2. The schedule and activities were overly ambitious. 3. A more focused approach, concentrating on a few areas and then branching out once accomplishments and benefits were well established, would have produced more sustainable outcomes. 4. The project had an overemphasis on construction – and not enough attention to other areas. 5. It is not enough to build and equip health care facilities – the facility utilization and perceptions of care by the target population are equally important in any attempt to increase access and quality.*

USAID/Washington funded efforts

Metro Manila Measles (HEALTHCOM Project) In activities around the world, this project's main goals were to use social marketing methods in communication aimed at encouraging health behaviour to reduce child mortality. Two main emphases were vaccination and treatment of diarrhoeal disease. A specific urban health activity took place in the Philippines; the EPI focused programme began with a pilot phase in Manila, then proceeded with a nationwide campaign.

The Metro Manila pilot began in 1988, using an integrated approach to assist the DOH in increasing vaccination coverage among children under one. Metro Manila is a large metropolitan area comprise 13 cities and municipalities. Manila was chosen because it had one of the lowest rates of full vaccination coverage in the country. The project worked with existing health services to increase outreach and user rates, upgrade health worker skills and disseminate health messages. Measles was the immunization focus because it was the most common childhood disease recognized by mothers, it was the third most common cause of death among infants and children in the Philippines, and because it was the final vaccination in the series, so it could catch children who had not received their other vaccinations (DPT, polio etc). From 1989 to 1990 a nationwide measles campaign was carried out in urban areas, growing out of the Manila campaign. Urban areas were the focus due to the fact that they had lower vaccination rates than rural areas (contrary to what many people had assumed).

The Philippines project was successful at increasing coverage and improving the timeliness of coverage – with different levels of success in different regions of the country.

> *Lessons learned: 1. It is critical to assess public awareness of the health problem to be targeted. 2. One must know the target audience. 3. Make the audience understand the benefit of adopting a health practice. 4. The communication team and collaborators must have a clear communication objective. 5. The team must use various communication channels. 6. The team needs a strong knowledge of health service delivery (logistics, policy, monitoring). 7. Assumptions about the needs and behaviour of urban populations, eg clinic hours being changed to accommodate working women, must be validated.*

WASH Project The Water and Sanitation for Health (WASH) Project was created in 1980 to provide technical assistance in water, sanitation and hygiene education to other development organizations under USAID's auspices. Designed to help the Agency address the 'water decade' of the 1980s, WASH began with a rural focus, but then reoriented its approach to address changing demographics. It was soon recognized that lessons learned in rural areas were not replicable in urban areas. The project carried out activities to seek new data sources and to compensate for the lack of data in urban areas, particularly those not included in any country's specific definition of urban. Although the project goal continued to be upgrading existing water supply and sanitation systems and developing replicable, self-sustaining new systems, added emphasis was placed on urban and solid waste issues.

> *Lessons learned: 1. The WASH Project has revealed some of the difficulties for a worldwide donor – those of facing different settings that require different approaches. 2. The project has found that 'a comprehensive interdisciplinary approach is needed [in urban sanitation], one that starts with seeking an understanding of the contextual issues: public health, environmental, social, financial, economic, legal, and institutional'. 3. Community ownership and involvement are crucial to sustainability, in urban areas as well as rural villages.*

The Resources for Child Health (REACH) Project conducted EPI activities in urban areas of Nigeria, Indonesia, Bangladesh, the Philippines, Turkey and Senegal. Some of these are described below.

National Urban EPI/Metropolitan Lagos Project An urban EPI effort was planned in Lagos, where, contrary to prior assumptions, urban coverage rates were especially low. Metropolitan Lagos has a population of over five million people, and is the largest urban metropolis in sub-Saharan Africa. The Nigerian government was spurred to action by the results of a study showing insufficient coverage in Lagos, especially for measles, and by the rapid spread of diseases in the country's urban areas. The government made immunization a priority. Under the project, REACH was to provide technical assistance to increase immunization coverage and sustainability in Lagos' 12 Local Government Areas (LGAs), and to devise models for programmes in other Nigerian cities. Immunization coverage surveys were carried out and analyzed, results were presented to government officials and used as baseline data.

> *Lessons learned: The project found a significant disparity between access and coverage (access was over 90 per cent in urban Lagos, but full immunization by age one ranged from 11 per cent to 41 per cent); and the strong role played by private sector providers – a role not previously recognized by either the national or local governments.*

Indonesia EPI project (1989–1990) REACH worked with the MOH to expand immunization through the National EPI. A major focus was expanding coverage in underserved urban populations, and determining reasons and solutions for the problem of lack of continuation to full immunization. REACH designed a social marketing study, conducted by a local social marketing research company; in Jakarta and Surabaya – the country's two largest cities – the data showed that the immunization effort had made progress: all except 7 per cent of babies were being at least partially immunized, and up to 55 per cent were fully immunized (representing progress over pre-project levels). After the social marketing work, REACH worked with the government to plan for expansion of urban EPI activities in Jakarta and Surabaya.

> **Lessons learned**: *The project found that in the following areas a specific urban focus was essential. 1. A need to target users and providers of immunization services. 2. Communication through appropriate and cost-effective mass media is needed to persuade mothers. 3. Service delivery difficulties need attention: training and absenteeism of providers, IEC, institutionalized followup procedures, free sample distribution, immunization cards, reaching the hard to reach urban poor (door to door, staff attitudes, offering incentives to mothers).*

REACH EPI activities also found that there were general areas of need in all of the urban settings where they conducted work in immunization programmes:

- Immunization delivery in urban settings is a great challenge that has not been addressed adequately. It is urgent that EPIs intensify urban efforts.
- Data on urban EPI are usually unavailable or unreliable. There is a need to collect essential indicators prior to interventions, and later to monitor these indicators as the activities progress in various city areas.
- The cultural and socio-economic heterogeneity of different parts of cities and peri-urban areas require tailored approaches.
- Epidemiology should guide strategies used in urban EPI efforts. Disease transmission patterns, roles of high-risk areas and groups, identification of areas of non-immunized children, roles of gathering places and seasonal migrations need to be quantified.
- Campaigns play an important role in urban settings: they increase awareness of the need for immunization and can interrupt disease transmission.

Lessons learned from other USAID health related efforts

USAID has also provided substantial support to PVOs working in urban health in several countries, through a competitive Child Survival grants programme. From 1985 to 1994, USAID committed $1.56 billion to Child Survival efforts in over 60 countries. Over 7 per cent of that ($110 million) was used to support efforts of PVOs through the Bureau for Humanitarian Response, Office of Private and Voluntary Cooperation. In fiscal year 1993, USAID's PVO Child Survival Programme supported 24 US PVOs engaged in 39 countries, and 17 of these projects were focused on urban areas. USAID recognizes the unique capabilities of PVOs in leveraging resources and providing services to population groups – including the urban poor – that the MOH often cannot reach. The Agency also understands PVOs' ability to establish good working relationships with the communities they serve making them effective in reaching especially vulnerable populations.

In September 1990 in Mexico City, an international 'Urban Lessons Learned' conference was held for USAID-supported PVOs working in urban areas. It was quickly recognized that:

> *the urban programmes were broader than the traditional child survival focus on childhood infectious disease seen in many rural programmes. Delegates were confronting problems common to the urban environment: contaminated bottle-feeding, substance abuse, HIV/AIDS, adolescent pregnancies, domestic violence, polluted water, piles of refuse, and smoke-laden air...In terms of management, PVOs identified more problems than solutions: volunteer turnover, high migration, overlapping agency responsibilities, and weak community participation where the sense of "community" was almost nonexistent. (Storms 1992 p2)*

A successor to the World Fertility Survey, the Demographic and Health Survey project (DHS) illustrates the difficulty of gathering data on the urban poor. Conducted in more than 35 countries around the world, DHS is a large USAID investment in data collection; yet given their national sampling, the ability to disaggregate data beyond urban and rural populations is close to impossible. Although attempts have been made to categorize respondents through correlations such as education, housing, water source and floor material of the home, and despite such a massive investment in data collection, the ability to obtain information on the urban poor is an approximation at best. [*Editors' note*: see *Child survival in big cities: are the poor disadvantaged?* by M. Brockerhoff, Population Council Working Paper number 58, 1993, for an analysis of urban DHS data.]

CURRENT STATUS OF URBAN HEALTH WITHIN USAID

United States development assistance is currently in a state of flux, due to belt-tightening throughout the US Government, new directions and changing events in foreign policy, and changing approaches within the development community. In addition, 'there is a growing inter-nationalization of traditionally national problems: AIDS, acid rain, the greenhouse effect, the ozone layer, environmental degradation, debt, narcotics, and urbanization... Many of them have their roots in poverty and rapid population growth' (Hamilton 1989 p28).

Changes for the Agency as a result of operating in the post Cold War environment can be seen in the 1994 *USAID Strategies for Sustainable Development*. Outside of efforts to reorganize the Agency, trim its ranks and make it more efficient, substantially limit the number of country missions, the goals of the long term efforts of USAID have been revised to be more relevant to the current realities. Support for sustainable and participatory development, collaboration and partnerships between host countries and donors, and the use of integrated approaches and methods – including the role of women – are cross cutting themes for all activities supported by the Agency. The categories of assistance fall into five categories:

1. protecting the environment;
2. building democracy;
3. stabilizing world population growth and protecting human health;

4. encouraging broad based economic growth;
5. providing humanitarian assistance and aiding post-crisis transitions.

Despite the many changes occurring within USAID, the Child Survival programme continues to be a focus for the Agency's Health and Nutrition Office.

> *At a time when resources are scarce and needs are great, building upon proven successes represents sound investment and wise policy. The Child Survival programme has the advantages of international consensus about what is needed, a proven track record, and demonstrated ability to learn from experience and adapt to changing circumstances. And, as a result of ongoing research, the programme will continue to provide the framework for introducing newly perfected technologies. (USAID 1992 p31)*

As noted previously, USAID staff are currently at a stage of discussion about the Agency's directions in the area of urban health. There is a great need for awareness raising within the agency and its cooperating agencies about the importance and needs of the urban poor. Interest in the topic appears to be on a slight increase, but Agency staff have not yet decided to focus on promoting the issue as one which USAID should build into its programmes.

Many of the critical issues in the urban health area fall under the five objectives of the Agency as mentioned above. Not only does improving the health of the poor in urban areas contribute to meeting objectives in all five areas, but it in fact surmounts prior programme and sectoral boundaries by its very nature of multisectoral coordination. In addition, working towards improved health of the urban poor necessitates a certain participation and effort by the communities involved – a highly regarded value of the Agency. Participatory development, the philosophy of accountability to the population being served, empowerment, and active community involvement and partnership is not only possible in the urban setting but is regarded to be one of the *most essential* components of any urban health activity.

There has, for several years, been a general understanding of the need for more cohesive urban development strategies in US economic assistance efforts. For example, the 1988–1989 Hamilton–Gilman congressional task force (through a study undertaken by Michigan State University) examined US foreign economic cooperation, and a priority area identified was: 'fostering sound urban development policies (especially given the fact that the majority of Third World poor will be urban residents within 20 years)' (Berg 1989 p32).

USAID does have an urban development policy, but the policy is for the Office of Housing and Urban Programmes, does not include other sectors involved in the issue and is not used by other Offices. 'Although AID has a written urban development policy, it is narrowly conceived and largely ignored...The policy determination is largely ignored by AID's regional bureaus...Thus, there is no effective coalition within the Agency to support programmes that explicitly address urban issues' (Rondinelli and Johnson 1990 pp260–261).

LOOKING TO THE FUTURE

First and foremost, USAID must define the issue and problems it faces in urban health, and decide upon its role and objectives in dealing with them. Then, it must devise a cohesive strategy for addressing the issue. This strategy must include specific elements for the Agency to focus on, targets and measures of progress and specific interventions for the Agency to undertake over time.

Prior to launching any new efforts targeted at the urban poor, the Agency must define the issue for itself – there must be acknowledgement of the problem within USAID and agreement that it is an appropriate problem for the Agency to address. To get officials to commit themselves to the issue, there is a need for a 'call to action' within USAID and the development community regarding the crisis of urban health and the need to act now to mitigate the certain problems of the future. There is a need to get USAID and other government officials to focus on the issue and understand its pervasiveness – USAID staff need to build a strong case to garner USAID (and congressional and Administration) support and interest in urban health.

USAID must then construct a framework for dealing with the issue of urban health – a conceptual structure of the issue to build it into USAID's diverse projects in various sectors. In defining the issue, USAID must recognize that it is broad based, that it is not a narrowly defined 'health' issue, 'population' issue, 'environmental' issue or 'economic' issue. Defining the issue requires a new way of looking at traditional USAID sectoral divisions and methods of economic assistance: this could be an opportune time for such reassessment by the Agency.

Several major positive aspects of working in cities can help USAID in devising and gaining support for an urban health strategy. In lobbying for the importance of such a strategy, USAID staff can draw parallels to the US domestic situation; can emphasize the potential for leveraging USAID's limited resources and gaining economies of scale in dense urban areas; can point to the relative ease of outreach and communication in cities and the advantages of the existing infrastructure there; can point to the large numbers of PVOs and NGOs (potential collaborators) located in cities; and can stress the proximity to policy makers and opinion leaders, who are usually based in capital cities. USAID can also point out the successes of its urban efforts to date, and the potential for the Agency to make a real difference in this area.

Critical problems in addressing urban health include first and foremost the lack of accurate data (and the lack of answers on how to obtain such data) on the urban poor, and differing definitions of what is 'urban'. The urban setting also offers the challenges of heterogeneous populations who are mobile and lacking clear constant social groupings, the necessity of working with different levels of government and the need to collaborate with private sector providers already working in cities (who are traditionally the least amenable to preventive and PHC approaches). In addition, USAID must overcome its longstanding rural bias and its relative lack of experience in urban work, and face the need to significantly restructure efforts to cross traditional sectoral boundaries.

The Agency must also address the difficulty of launching new efforts with shrinking resources and closing missions (and a Congress responding to the American public's calls to do more about domestic problems and reluctant to spend more tax dollars on foreign assistance.)

USAID has certain comparative advantages in approaching the complex issue of urban health. These include the following:

- strength in information/education/communication (IEC) campaigns, and a proven history in this area;
- an understanding of the private sector, how to work with it and the need for its cooperation;
- potential for coordinated Agency efforts, with collaboration among USAID Washington, missions and regional offices (although worldwide representation will diminish somewhat with the closing of some USAID missions);
- a willingness to make investments and experiment with innovative approaches without clear outcomes; and built-in project flexibility to adapt to local situations;
- visibility and experience in technical assistance and policy reform;
- a focus on sustainable and participatory development;
- science and technology and education expertise;
- Office of Housing and Urban Programmes experience working with local governments and municipalities.

In contrast, USAID has certain constraints to working successfully on new, targeted urban health initiatives. These include

- a proclivity to work with MOH level officials, and lack of significant Agency experience working with municipal governments with the exception of the Office of Housing and Urban Programmes;
- a division within the Agency between the Health Office and the Office of Housing and Urban Programmes which could hinder urban health efforts (although this division should improve with Agency restructuring);
- apportionment of foreign aid funds and current budget cuts do not leave room for new investments;
- current uncertainty and low morale in the Agency over its upheaval, restructuring and downsizing; and
- a lack of coordination among USAID efforts at the central level although coordination and collaboration among sectors tends to occur in the field.

The following are the basic necessary elements of an urban health strategy for the Agency:

- **Vision** USAID first and foremost requires an urban health 'vision' of what the problem is about and what the Agency can bring to bear on the issue to unify staff behind a common general theme. This vision would include an internal Agency urban health strategy, and a vision of what should happen in projects in the field.
- **Objectives** USAID needs to set some clear objectives which are

quantifiable to be used as specific roadmarkers. These objectives must be clear, focused, measurable, realistic, and should serve as guides for activities in the years to come. Objectives should be delineated in two sets: long term, more general urban health objectives; and short term, specific objectives in order to ensure concrete progress.

- **Activities** Following the established vision and objectives, USAID must develop specific urban health activities (both long-term and short-term).

- **Workplan** Once activities have been decided upon, USAID must then establish a workplan for getting them done. This plan organizes activities in order of priority and by taking into account considerations of time, staff and funding. Each activity must be given a budget, including realistic assessments of necessary time and staff. USAID's urban health workplan can be done in three levels: a general plan for the coming five years; a specific first year plan; and a very detailed plan for the first three months.

- **Monitoring progress** USAID may wish to establish an urban health task force to oversee and monitor implementation of urban health activities by centrally funded and bilateral projects. Such a monitoring group could monitor progress quarterly and draft the workplan for the next quarter. This group would work to ensure consistency, effectiveness and efficiency among the Agency's various urban health efforts.

CONCLUSIONS

As the Agency stated in its 1993 Congressional Presentation:

> *AID is facing a complex and challenging task over the next few years, adjusting to new programme priorities to meet the post Cold War realities, addressing accountability and management issues and, at the same time, reducing the cost of operating the Agency. To accomplish this, AID will: 1) cease doing some things that are now being done; 2) do other things in different and less staff-intensive ways; and 3) operate with fewer staff, both overseas and in Washington. (USAID 1993a p15)*

With the current situation, the reality is that it will be extremely difficult for Agency staff to launch any new initiative such as a focus on urban health. Perhaps the most that can be done in the short term is to raise consciousness about the issue in USAID and the Congress and make urban health an integral component of existing initiatives.

USAID's future efforts in urban health will not likely entail new projects with an urban health focus, especially within the current and foreseeable future of limited budgets. Instead, efforts can be built into existing or newly awarded projects in various sectors, which will adapt and seek new ways to meet the needs of the neglected urban poor. The challenge will be to have a unified USAID-wide strategy and approach implemented in a coordinated way by the various relevant projects under various USAID offices. USAID does have experience with integration of efforts across sectoral areas: 'AID integrates environmental concerns across development sectors. Environmental activities are included in programmes such as trade and investment, agriculture, health and education, as well as in purely environmental projects' (USAID 1993b p7). Institutionalization of gender concerns is another area in which USAID has worked to integrate activities across sectors and encourage collaboration among relevant technical areas.

USAID has the opportunity to take the lead on the issue of urban health, to try new ways of addressing development challenges, change with the times and prepare for the future. The Agency can attempt new types of initiatives in integrating sectoral efforts to improve the overall conditions and health of the urban poor. Urban health is a relatively new focus area, one in which there are not yet many actors. USAID could take a proactive stance and encourage other donors to follow. In this era of belt-tightening and budget cuts (and USAID reorganization), greater efficiency, collaboration with other institutions and intersectoral cooperation could be natural, positive results of the need to maximize the impact of limited resources.

USAID's current situation of upheaval and reorganization is only a small part of the Agency's overall situation. USAID staff must attempt to look beyond the immediate uncertainty of budgets, staffing levels, and organizational structures, and think about development challenges of the future – including urban health – and the likely role of the US Agency for International Development into the next century.

AID needs a concerted strategy to address urban issues if it is to respond more effectively to the changing characteristics of its clientele and to the pervasive impacts of urbanization during the 1990s. A strategy is needed because most of the problems and opportunities arising from rapid urbanization cross AID's sectoral and programme boundaries... Without an urban strategy AID is likely to incur serious opportunity costs in planning programmes and allocating resources during the 1990s. (Rondinelli and Johnson 1990 pp259–260)

REFERENCES

Berg, R (1989) The United States and the Majority of the Third World *Foreign Service Journal*, February, pp32–33

Bissell, R (1989) Back to the Drafting Table *Foreign Service Journal*, February, pp34–38

Hamilton, L (1989) Foreign Assistance: Which Direction Now? *Foreign Service Journal*, February, pp27–31

Rondinelli, D and Johnson, R (1990) Third World Urbanization and American Foreign Policy: Development Assistance in the 1990's *Policy Studies Review*, vol 9 no 2, pp246–262

Storms, D (ed) (1992) *Report from the Cities: Cases in Urban Child Survival Management PVO Child Survival Programme 1985–1992* Institute for International Programmes, School of Hygiene and Public Health, The Johns Hopkins University, Baltimore

USAID (1982) *AID Policy Paper: Health Assistance*

USAID (1992) *Child Survival: A Seventh Report to Congress on the USAID Programme*

USAID (1993a) *Congressional Presentation Fiscal Year 1994*

USAID (1993b) *Child Survival: An Eighth Report to Congress on the USAID Programme*

11

A Decade of GTZ's Experience in Urban Health

Fred Merkle and Uli Knobloch

'HEALTH FOR ALL' – THE RURAL BIAS

During the 1960s and 1970s 'Health in the Cities' was a rather neglected issue. Concepts and strategies for 'Health for All' concentrated on rural health systems, and primary health care (PHC) was mainly based on the fundamental needs perceived by those responsible for rural health systems, and the participation of rural communities. This bias towards rural development was maintained by international and bilateral donor agencies because of several misleading perceptions:

- Urban statistics for health in relation to population look better than rural ones. This is a result of averaging data for the rich and poor, and of the lack of health data for the poorest.
- The sophisticated and expensive infrastructures which consume most resources are situated in the cities. However, they serve only a minority of the population, and an even smaller proportion of those most in need.
- Rural development programmes were expected to reduce migration to the cities. This did not, in fact, happen.
- In a situation in which economic progress was given pride of place the health impact of industrialization, modernization and uncontrolled growth was not recognized.

During the 1980s it was realized that these perceptions of the health situation in cities did not reflect reality. One third of the people in Africa are living in cities, and in Latin America around two thirds, and most of these city dwellers are very poor and do not have access to health and social services. In many development agencies, including those under the German government (like GTZ, KfW, DSE etc) this recognition has induced a shift in policy. Whereas until now more than two thirds of aid funds were still used for rural projects, an increasing proportion is now directed towards urban development including health.

Since 1980 the German Agency for Technical Cooperation (GTZ) has planned and implemented more than ten pilot projects on behalf of the German government in the sector of 'Health, Population and Nutrition', and approximately 100 in health related sectors (eg water, waste disposal etc). The mandate of GTZ is presented in Box 11.1.

What are the reasons for this change in attitude?

- In the early 1980s many requests from developing countries for structural improvement in cities (transportation, housing, water, sanitation etc) reached the German government. In the process of their appraisal it became clear that the existing intra-urban differences (including health) are not just functions of structures but effects of socio-economic conditions and political priority setting.
- There was an increasing understanding that economic growth depends on educated and healthy people in urban as well as in rural areas.
- The idea that concentration on rural development and poverty alleviation in rural areas would keep more people in the countryside was not successful:
  - Investments through bilateral cooperation were insufficient to level out existing imbalances in trade, employment opportunities and social investments from the governments; because of this, it was not possible to create multiple smaller urban growth centres throughout countries, which could reduce migration to capital cities.
  - It became clear that modernization of agriculture usually leads to less labour intensive procedures ie to higher rural unemployment.
  - Better education facilities in the cities are attracting a lot of adolescents from the countryside who tend to search for any income opportunities rather than return to their families.
- It became clear that political stability and even the fate of governments is mostly determined by socio-economic factors affecting the life of urban citizens, including the poor.

First project experiences showed that approaches developed for rural health programmes cannot be applied under urban conditions. Research on urban health development was an area in which remarkably little work had been done until the mid-1980s. Therefore understanding of the factors that determine 'well-being' in the city, and of priority needs, and the causes of disease, is still very limited.

UNDERSTANDING THE DETERMINANTS OF URBAN HEALTH

The complex and dynamic social structures and extreme income differences within cities are not suitable for simple approaches. Most large cities can be divided into four types of areas with basically different settings:

Box 11.1

THE MANDATE OF GTZ

The mandate of GTZ, the German Agency for Technical Cooperation, is to concentrate on the development of human resources and local institutions by support of training, research and appropriate strategies. The agency is mainly funded by the German government and follows the agreed priorities and policy guidelines for development cooperation:

- poverty alleviation and security of basic needs;
- sustainable development through appropriate and ecologically sound strategies;
- strengthening of local capacities (including the role of women).

In the sector of Health, Population and Nutrition there are approximately 120 projects in more than 50 countries under implementation. About 10 per cent of them are concentrating on issues of urban health; this share is, however, expected to increase over the coming years. The sector deals with about 8 per cent of the government allocation for technical cooperation,

---

1. **Old central part** with a high population concentration, frequently with decaying buildings and outdated services, and often used for 'grey markets'.
2. **Planned middle class area** with moderate population density, adequate services and functioning infrastructure.
3. **Prosperous elite area** with a low population density, all services, sophisticated infrastructure and business establishments.
4. **Peri-urban areas** undefined, densely populated, mixed with industries, fast growth (approximately 70 per cent of the new migrants). The population of these peri-urban areas can be divided into three different categories: those living in legally accepted settlements, illegal squatters and floating population.

Whereas historically most cities were built and developed in the ecologically most suitable environment, many slums are developing in marginal areas of cities like garbage dumping sites, steep hills, seasides or the banks of creeks etc. In these situations people are exposed to natural disasters, and it is extremely difficult to provide the necessary infrastructures like roads, water and sewer systems.

In discussing urban areas we have to keep in mind that we are usually dealing with these four settings, which create forces of attraction and also acute tensions within the cities. People from outside, particularly from the countryside, are attracted to the cities by settings of the second and third types, but mostly end up in the fourth type of areas. People in settings two and three will generally try to prevent the entrance of the people from setting four into their areas. But the four settings are in no way fixed or stagnant; they are constantly undergoing an uncontrollable dynamic development.

In many cities, poor people in peri-urban areas make up more than half of the population. According to our experience, surveys and social

programmes mostly reach the first category of the poor, in the stable settlements. Illegal squatters and floating groups are left out as far as health information systems are concerned, and remain at the periphery of most intervention programmes. For most of the migrants coming into the cities, economic reasons are the most important:

- The low productivity or even deterioration of rural economies (increased by a disproportionately high population growth) can be considered as a 'push factor'.
- Even if people have no clear prospect of employment nor a place to live, the productivity and the better infrastructure of the cities – things like roads, electricity, communication and entertainment act as strong 'pull factors'.

There is no question that for most developing countries only increased productivity in the modern sector (ie industry and services) can solve the increasing economic dilemma, but most countries have failed to decentralize modern production into many smaller 'growth centres' across the country. As an extreme result, we can see conglomerations like Mexico City, São Paulo or, in the ASEAN region, Bangkok, where 10 per cent of the national population produces 80 per cent of Thailand's GNP. However, even with this increased productivity the cities cannot absorb or employ the millions of migrants from rural areas (which is probably the most significant difference from the urbanization in Europe). The bulk of migrants are left fighting for survival by taking opportunistic jobs in the so called 'grey market'. Without their cheap labour large sectors in production and services in the cities could not exist. In this situation, poor people in urban areas have to venture into any area of income generation that is available. Considerations about safety and health related risks at the workplace or at home will be given second priority.

It is obvious that the traditional aid agency priorities of tropical medicine and public health are no longer appropriate. Epidemiological models of transmission, with vectors, agents and infected persons, are only partly applicable in an urban slum in which, besides infection, there is a multiplicity of psychosocial, nutritional and toxic determinants of illness (see the chapter by Seager).

Three characteristics of urban economic growth affect health and social well-being more than others:

1. **Environmental hazards and the toxic wastes** These are present at the workplace, at home and everywhere else in the city, and very often even spill over into rural areas. They probably cause more damage to health than infectious diseases. Leading causes for diseases among the urban poor are:
   - inadequate disposal of solid waste;
   - lack of an adequate and safe water supply;
   - insanitary disposal of excreta;
   - inadequate housing and domestic hygiene;
   - exposure to toxic and caustic substances including pollution;
   - poor food safety;
   - social and mental stress.

2. **The socio-economic differences** Cities house the richest and the poorest. Extreme luxury and deepest misery may be found within the same vicinity. This extreme discrepancy is also reflected in services, including health.
3. **Unplanned growth** City administrations have been unable to cope with the unplanned growth and have lost control over large parts of the cities. Existing laws and regulations are bypassed, and city planning is influenced by groups with particular economic interests and with the financial means to manipulate political decisions.

DISEASES, GROUPS AT RISK AND SERVICES

Diseases

Health surveys among the urban poor – despite their limited coverage - reflect the changes in their lifestyle and their environment. There are many variations between different cities, but the following results from a baseline survey in Cúcuta, Colombia (see Box 11.2) and from surveys in Manila indicate some trends. Accidents, homicides and suicides frequently become the leading causes of death. Morbidity is marked by accidents and violence, diseases associated with sexual behaviour (including AIDS, which is mostly an urban disease), drug and alcohol abuse and psychosocial problems. Chronic problems due to air and food can only be guessed at. At the same time, some infectious diseases such as diarrhoea, ARI, tuberculosis and dengue are more prevalent in slum areas. Cardiovascular diseases and neoplasms are increasing among people moving from rural areas to Third World cities. This situation thus demonstrates how the urban poor can be caught in a stage of epidemiological transition, with a high risk for both 'traditional' infectious diseases, and 'modern' ones.

A nutrition survey for low income groups (Cúcuta baseline survey) showed the changes in lifestyle and risks resulting from urban living:

• a greater diversity of foods but almost complete reliance on purchases of cheap food, leading to problems if prices fluctuate and income decreases;
• uncertain risks from street food;
• earlier and inadequate supplementary feeding with substitution of infant formula or diluted milk for breastfeeding;
• 80 per cent of children (12–24 months) receive only three or fewer meals a day;
• high prevalence of diarrhoeal disease (approximately 20 per cent in children under five years old).

Groups at risk

Women often suffer most from socioeconomic conditions in cities. In many cases, the mother is the sole support of the family, and women suffer from many discriminatory economic and social practices, including prostitution. 'Conventional' health services concentrate on mother and child health (MCH), and give little attention to economic and social problems of women, for example, working conditions in factories, maltreatment, drug dependence etc. The absence or unavailability of effective family planning methods contributes not only to the growth of urban slums, but also to unplanned pregnancies, high abortion rates and high maternal mortality. Last but not least, the unavailability of condoms contributes to the spread of STDs and AIDS.

Experience shows that only a minor proportion of women in need are seen at the health centres in the city. The challenge remains to provide basic health and family planning services including social counselling near the workplaces or living quarters, at a time when the women can attend, for example, mothers' groups in the evenings.

Children and adolescents must be seen as another group at risk – both immediate and long term. Often growing up without parents and homes, they are sometimes forced into the labour market at an early age. Many of them become petty criminals, pursued both by the law and criminal gangs, or are exploited and forced into servitude and prostitution. Adolescents are in great need of effective guidance on health behaviour, but are seldom reached by established health services.

Health services

In many cities, some health and family planning services or drug supplies are within easy reach of the poor, but even in these cases open or hidden charges and unsatisfactory services hinder their actual use. Many slum quarters do not have any health centres at all. The ability of urban health services to influence health related behaviour, and to motivate local politicians and administrators to invest more in water, sanitation and pollution control is very limited.

PHC FOR AND WITH THE URBAN POOR

The foregoing analysis of the situation of urban health in developing countries does not attempt to be comprehensive. It summarizes results of baseline studies, pilot and research projects and workshops organized by GTZ. The findings are not necessarily generalizable – each city has its own environment, with specific socio-economic conditions and causes of illness, and its own pattern of available services. They have, however, urged us to rethink conventional approaches to improving health. A relevant experience of GTZ is presented in Box 11.2.

As a first step, in order to understand the physiology and pathophysiology of the 'urban body', with its interdependent organs and functions, we have to invest more into research: baseline surveys in typical groups and communities; and inventories of existing services, institutions and programmes.

The involvement of local universities with their young and socially motivated staff can be useful to identify appropriate and innovative strategies, to generate an increased awareness of urban problems and to develop skills in conducting urban field research. We see this as an important contribution to more meaningful 'essential national health research'.

Box 11.2

PROJECT EXAMPLE: PHC IN MARGINAL URBAN AREAS OF CÚCUTA, COLOMBIA

Executing agencies: Servicio Seccional de salud de norte de Santander NORSSALUD and GTZ

Project period: 1988–1994, planned extension 1995–1997

Budget (projected) 6.4 million DM

Project Area: Metropolitan area of Cúcuta (including Los Patios)

Target population: Low income areas of Atalaya, Northern Area and Los Patios, approximately 200,000 inhabitants

Project goal: To contribute to the improvement of the health situation in low income urban areas of Cúcuta

Project objective: To elaborate and to test strategies and replicable components (modules) for the implementation of primary health care concept in poor urban areas

The four main working areas are:
– strengthening of management capacity of the local health systems;
– reinforcement of local health services with innovative contents and approaches;
– improvement of basic environmental conditions (water, sanitation, solid waste);
– strengthening community participation.

Difficulties:
– Only few investments in the social sector.
– Process of decentralization very slow, almost resistance against the change, therefore no coherent urban health infrastructure.
– Lack of institutional personnel, like social workers (especially for 'extramural' community activities).
– Decisions of health authorities often politically and not technically influenced.
– Low motivation of health personnel in the government health centres (bad pay, few incentives) produces poor quality of services and under-utilization.
– Lack of adequate supervision.

After four years of execution some promising results have been achieved:
– Social privatization of municipal **waste collection** and transport with good cost efficiency as well as creation of new independent jobs and decrease of environmental risks. Rotation funds permit replication without external support.
– Improvement of sanitary conditions with the **'Healthy House' concept** with its educative, technical and economic components and participatory elements (people pay for materials and installations or construct themselves) which contributes to a healthier environment and promotes a solution by the people themselves.
– Improvement of **low cost drugs** accessibility through community enterprises (cooperative systems) with autonomous administration and technical supervision by the health sector. The two existing cooperatives are already financially completely independent and maintain themselves.

- The **home and community gardens** which represent a potential to improve nutrition and to generate income for poor urban households.
- The community based **oral rehydration units** which contribute to reduce the complications of diarrhoeal disease especially in small children.
- The **Community Health Schools** as an instrument for community based health education and health promotion.
- The improvement of peripheral **health centres'** infrastructure with delivery rooms, observation wards, laboratories and dentistry units as well as necessary equipment in order to prevent congestion of the regional hospital with low risk patients.
- The procurement of necessary equipment for the departmental public health laboratory.
- The strengthening of the **referral system** by means of a radio-communication system between the regional hospital and the peripheral health units.
- The improvement of the **managerial capacity within the local institutions**.
- The development of a **local research unit** to support research activities for planning, evaluating and decision making processes.

Types of studies carried out:
- Nutrition and Health baseline survey
- Study of morbidity and utilization of health services
- KAP study on water and sanitation
- Study about intestinal parasitism
- KAP study about dengue
- Study of quality of health services for women
- Study about management of hospital waste

In general, the project succeeded in coordinating efforts of various different institutions (governmental and nongovernmental) to cooperate in health related aspects and social development in the municipalities of Cúcuta and Los Patios. The question is whether these achievements can be maintained without a 'catalyst-agency' after the project's 'lifetime'. On the other hand, the dynamics of self-administered autonomous processes and new types of community organizations are very promising with regard to sustainability. The programme succeeded in integrating fully measures to improve the environment into the health project, which is fundamental for improving health and quality of life in urban low income areas.

The principles underlying primary health care were described in the Declaration of Alma Ata as a set of seven elements. In the attempt to create better health conditions in the cities, however, PHC has to be seen even more as a social movement. Community action needs to be promoted and supported on a much larger scale.

With the dwindling influence of governments on city planning and management, effective community organizations are needed more than ever. In most urban settings, such organizations and concerned groups already exist; these groups should be offered external support to help them to grow into functional community organizations and political pressure groups.

The role of the government health and family planning services may often be limited by their traditional sectoral orientation and by loyalty to the ruling political power. In order to mobilize communities, to link them with different governmental and Non-governmental organizations, and to plan and to implement activities for priority needs (which might not be health services related), a new breed of 'social facilitator' is needed. Ideally, such people should be full time salaried workers, and they should be independent for better credibility.

In many depressed urban areas, communities can hardly be defined, for lack of geographical distinction and a lack of developed organizational structures or leadership. But in most instances, groups can be identified which have a common concern around certain priority problems. Guidance in conducting a community diagnosis, which leads to an understanding of the causes and effects of the problem, can lead to plan of action. Peer groups and informal leadership will develop around such a common cause. The community volunteers emerging from such systems have in many instances gone on to become local political leaders.

Community oriented services should meet their clientele in the districts where they live, and work with local groups on their particular health problems. Often this process creates approaches that are new for these areas; in health care and family planning services, for example:

- evening clinics for working women;
- day care centres for children;
- drug cooperatives and treatment centres for diarrhoea;
- beauty parlours with STD and AIDS counselling.

However, community based activities cannot be restricted to health issues alone. They have to include perceived priority needs like income generation or housing.

When **external support** is offered, it should be done with the objective of enabling local groups/communities to solve their problems, and turning apathy or resignation into social action. Laws and regulations – which will be evaded or even force people into criminality – are less effective than support and incentives to develop a healthier environment. People who are given secured land tenure will improve their housing with all available resources. If they have access to favourable credits and to building materials they will make further improvements. There have been encouraging examples where community actions were able to improve local water supply, drainage and waste disposal.

Health programmes in cities have to become much more intersectoral. Agencies in charge of city planning, housing, industries, water sanitation, transportation, education, entertainment and sport and many other sectors, contribute to making cities healthier. A multiplicity of government and private health service facilities often exist, and there are frequently numerous NGOs with different interests all acting independently. The success of city health programmes depends to a large extent on the insight that the programme managers have into this network, and their ability to mobilize the different actors in an orchestrated way.

Experience in our projects, and in the WHO 'Healthy Cities' programme (see the chapter by Goldstein et al), also shows that much can be achieved by convincing heads and members of local governments about the political importance of the concept, making them the 'prime mover' in the health programme.

Governments cannot be released from their basic responsibility for carrying out city planning and management so as to ensure a health promoting environment. One of their responsibilities is the prevention of industrial and domestic pollution. In this area, a much stricter monitoring and enforcement of laws is needed. The important role of street food in many places as a nutritional basis of the poor requires education of vendors and the establishment and monitoring of hygiene standards.

Community oriented health services must find a new role in the cities. They can increase their influence in creating a 'healthier city' by means of:

- intensive and innovative health education to reach groups at risk: eg with programmes for school and street children, youth, personnel and clients of the entertainment industry etc;
- supporting community oriented and need based programmes as discussed above;
- analysis of health problems resulting from manmade environmental and occupational hazards;
- advocacy for health among intersectoral and political groups (eg city councils);
- provision of a basic referral system for sick people at a cost the poor can afford.

With the changing disease pattern in cities, we have to reorient approaches towards better health. One of these newly-emerging strategies is 'Primary Environmental Care'. This is a process by which individuals and communities learn to understand the effects of manmade environment (in public, at home and at the workplace) and to develop responsibility for environmental care. At the same time, the fulfilment of basic needs (including health, education and income) should be assured.

City development has to be understood as a process in which both rural and urban people are affected. We must see it as the most critical determinant for the future in each country. Economic survival and progress, social peace and political stability of a country will primarily depend on people living in and around cities. It is the challenge of the 1990s to find ways and means to involve them in a social development process, and to secure their basic human needs including health care.

12

Non-governmental Organizations – at the Interface between Municipalities and Communities

Sarah J Atkinson (ed)

**Based on contributions by Doreen Gihanga, Quazi Ghiasuddin
(SCF-UK) , and Katherine Kaye (formerly SC, USA)**

INTRODUCTION

Non-governmental organizations (NGOs) are becoming increasingly important as players in development activities. Recent estimates are of more than 2000 NGOs from the OECD countries, working with up to 20,000 southern based NGOs (Clark 1990). The numbers reported indicate the diverse roles and activities carried out by agencies collectively labelled as NGOs. Classifications of NGOs have distinguished organizations according to where they are based and the kinds of activities in which they are involved (Clark 1990, Edwards and Hulme 1992).

This paper will focus on the role of international NGOs in urban health by presenting case examples of work, approaches, advantages and constraints from two comparable international organizations: Save the Children USA (SC US) and Save the Children Fund UK (SCF UK).

The strength of NGOs has long been recognized as lying in the local nature of their actions, the relationships they establish, their flexibility in managing projects and responding to local circumstances and the values with which they work. NGOs often work in establishing community based projects and in bridging the relationship between communities or community based organizations and the local or national government. However, although NGOs may have great impact locally on the lives of people, the extent of their impact is limited and does not usually address the structures and processes which determine resource distribution internationally, nationally or even within a region. How NGOs can improve the impact of their developmental activities has become a concern of many international agencies. Edwards and Hulme (1992) state that the central question for NGOs of all kinds is how can they increase their developmental impact without losing their traditional flexibility, value base and effectiveness at the local level?

In contrast to NGOs, governments have the systems and structures to reach many people but usually have a small impact. NGOs are sometimes seen by international donors as an effective and efficient channel for development funds and programme management. At the same time, since national NGOs and southern counterpart NGOs are becoming increasingly strong, the appropriate role for international NGOs might be rather one of advocacy to governments both in the South and in the North and to other international agencies. Practical questions for international NGOs regarding improving impact are how international NGOs can and should work with governments, to what extent they should accept contracts to deliver development programmes from bilateral and multilateral agencies and how they maintain their legitimacy to speak for the poorest to the international community when their activities at local level have decreased.

In the health sector, NGOs have typically been great supporters and proponents of the primary health care (PHC) approach. For example, the policy for health activities of SCF UK includes a statement, 'SCF works firmly within the context of the Alma Ata declaration on primary health care' (Save The Children Fund UK 1992). The two agencies represented in this chapter are typical of international NGOs working in health in having a long experience of implementing PHC in rural areas. As more attention is given to the need for basic health care in urban areas, the NGO community are well placed to assess the appropriateness of their rural experience for urban areas.

The rest of the chapter will present examples of three projects in urban areas run by the two international NGOs. Three themes related to the role of NGOs in urban health are raised by the examples:

1. Working with urban communities to establish participatory urban primary health care.
2. Reviewing the appropriateness of rural experiences for urban areas and the extent that adaptation or new approaches are needed.
3. Strategies for scaling-up and increasing impact of NGO projects in urban areas.

SAVE THE CHILDREN FUND UK

Save the Children Fund UK (SCF UK) have supported the primary health care approach since the Alma Ata declaration. A summary of the SCF UK health sector policy (Save the Children Fund UK 1992) demonstrates the combination of traditional NGO values, some ambivalences arising from the modified role of international NGOs in the 1990s and indicates strategies for a wider developmental impact.

The health sector policy of SCF UK has the following main points:

• Support to the implementation of national health sector policies which are characterized by appropriateness, universal availability, community participation, particularly where these relate to mother and child health.

- Provision of support only where this can be sustained through the financial, organizational and other constraints of the countries and communities and provision of health services directly only in exceptional circumstances such as for displaced populations and although not imposing conditions on the provision of support, will seek to influence policy through partnership with government and communities.
- Support given to any level or type of activity which is of fundamental importance to the development of national health services, involves an advisory role nationally or regionally and which builds on SCF's experience in that country so that assistance is provided competently and effectively.
- Experience gained from its overseas projects will be used to influence the international community involved in the health sector.
- Support for cost sharing will be given only where it is compatible with equity in service delivery and SCF will not to work directly with the commercial health sector where the aim is profit rather than universal service provision.

SCF UK builds up long-term working relationships in countries over many years. The development of specific projects in any field has an *ad hoc* element in so far as the NGO can react to issues as they emerge locally through negotiation with government and other agencies. Two examples of SCF UK projects demonstrate how an NGO can work in primary health care in urban areas. The first supports rehabilitation and provision of basic health care in Kampala, Uganda, ensuring impact by influencing policymaking as well as having specific inputs on a wide scale. The second project is developing district level models for health care which can be exported to other districts across the city in Khulna, Bangladesh.

Health service provision in Kampala City Council
(Based on information from Doreen Gihanga)

Health care in Kampala was originally designed in the 1970s to serve a total city population of around 300,000. The following years have been marked by continual civil strife. The population of Kampala has grown dramatically over this time from rapid migration of populations from war areas and from internal growth, to an estimated population of over one million. The civil war brought with it economic recession, an increase in poverty and associated ill health together with deterioration in public services, such as health care. As the population grew, the limited health care available through the health clinics became inaccessible since the health centres are concentrated in the original centre of the city. In any case, the health clinics do not have adequate capacity to cope with the current population size. The city has seven clinics of which two are for the City Council staff and their families. The Kampala city general population therefore has access to only five clinics. Urban residents seeking formal health care use private practitioners if they can afford to do so or go directly to the main government hospital (Mulago hospital).

As a result of the lack of alternative public health centres, the hospital is severely overcrowded and figures of up to 50 per cent more patients than beds have been reported.

Since the current government came to power, ending the national civil war, the Kampala City Council has started to review health care in the city and to rehabilitate the network of government services. A primary health care model has been adopted in the country, although the experience of implementing this approach has largely been rural. The first step is to rehabilitate the existing health clinics in terms of both physical structure and available health personnel in order to decrease the demand for deliveries and both curative and preventive care at the hospital outpatients department.

SCF UK has agreed to support the City Council with the rehabilitation of health clinics and establishment of primary health care in Kampala. NGOs are particularly well placed to assist governments with building up or rehabilitating urban health systems given their local level of operations which enables a rapid and largely informal mechanism of feedback on the success or otherwise of measures. NGOs have been active in primary health care approaches for local health systems and community participation in Uganda for many years in rural areas. The translation of that experience to urban areas demonstrates the heterogeneity of city districts in that the approaches were successful in some areas but need to be reassessed and adapted for other districts. Working closely with the government enhances the potential impact of the NGO's local level activities. In the case of Kampala, the NGO focused on certain activities within the provision of primary health care in all five clinics, thus having a potential impact on a large population.

The SCF UK inputs into the establishment of primary health care in Kampala operate at two levels: the clinic and the community. The first inputs have been assistance to physical and human resources to rehabilitate the clinics, with particular emphasis on mother and child health (MCH) services. Following this, MCH activities were initiated in the community through community health workers, trained birth attendants and women's support groups. The community based activities initially focused on antenatal care, family planning, child health and nutrition education. SCF UK started working in Kampala in 1985 with three of the clinics and later expanded to all five.

By 1993, SCF UK could report that its original objectives for supporting the rehabilitation of clinics had largely been achieved. All the clinics are now functioning well, providing MCH services as planned in the project design. The improvement in both quality and quantity of services provided is reflected in the increased attendance seen at the clinics.

Problems of course remain for the provision of primary health care in Kampala. There are still only the five original clinics so access is still difficult from peri-urban areas. The salaries for public health workers and health officers in the City Council are low. As a result, many staff are leaving the public sector in favour of the private sector which is causing a serious shortage of staff, especially of midwives. Those remaining are too few, overworked and thus badly demoralized. Needless to say, under such conditions the quality of care provided is often poor. The City

Council is responsible for repairs and maintenance of all the structures in the city including health facilities. However, since the health department has not historically generated any of its own funds, funding is dependent on the allocation to health from the City Council budget. Health is not the city's first priority and the health department is usually only allocated a small budget. Moreover, the official budget allocated for health may sometimes not be released.

Although the initial objectives of the project were clinic based rather than community based, once the first phase of physical rehabilitation was underway and the clinics running, the need to complement the clinic services with some community based health activities emerged. The clinics were only providing a limited package of services at this stage and therefore mother support groups were started in the community to discuss other issues such as nutrition and hygiene in the home.

The main SCF UK inputs have been establishing mother support groups, training community health workers (mostly women) and traditional birth attendants (all women). The project is currently establishing local community councils, called village health communities, which will help the City Council to run the clinics and through which it is hoped to increase the participation of the community.

The idea for mother support groups followed the successful experience of this kind of initiative in one area of Kampala, Kawempe. Two more mother support groups were then started in two other areas of Kampala. The initial objective was to improve child survival through support, promotion and protection for breastfeeding. The attendance was good and soon mothers started asking questions regarding other health issues such as AIDS, nutrition, immunization and family planning. It was then decided to meet once a month to discuss a topic chosen by the group beforehand. The NGO would try to bring along someone working in the field to lead the group discussion and answer specific questions. The women have become knowledgeable about many diseases, their causes and prevention. The women are keen to put into practice the discussions of prevention and the health workers see this happening when they make home visits. The community health workers are members of the support group voluntarily, indicating their commitment to their work and eagerness to pass on information they have received through training.

As an unplanned benefit, the group has helped women get to know each other very well and also to discover skills amongst group members. The group has started producing handicrafts with those experienced in this work teaching those previously unskilled.

The establishment of a village health committee will provide a link between the government health authority and the local community. The government now supports and encourages community participation. Through the village health committee, the community will be able to identify their health problems, establish priorities and find appropriate solutions. The village health committees have a strong foundation emerging from the system of grass roots based Resistance Councils established by the present government in which all individuals are encouraged to get involved and participate in all decisions regarding development.

A number of urban specific problems to be tackled have emerged from the initial community based activities, mainly regarding the constraints on participation in an urban setting.

Accommodation in peri-urban areas is scarce and of extremely poor quality. Urban residents in the poor areas of the city rent their houses and are therefore not free to improve the structure or add other structures on the land such as latrines or racks for drying household utensils or compost pits for refuse disposal. The people are unable to approach the landlord to ask about improving the site, since the landlords often only appear every six months simply to collect the rent. Most of the group activities such as the health eduction and women support groups take place outside working hours, often on Sundays. One person is usually selected to lead the group, but if the discussion leader fails to turn up, the group loses morale very quickly and may not attend the next meeting. Those involved in community based activities want some form of incentive. The dependency on a cash economy in the city means any time given to community activities is at the cost of potential earnings. In response to this, the project has started up some income generating activities. The Kampala City Council welfare department has also been approached for support to the groups and to the community.

The model adopted is similar to the rural experience of primary health care in which a health centre offering basic health care is embedded in and works closely with the local, residential community. In two of the clinic areas (Kawempe and Kisenyi), this approach has been very successful and the experience reported above of the community based activities are mainly taken from these two. In these areas, the population is permanent, people are of the same culture and speak the same language. However, this is not the case for the majority of the clinics, that is three out of the five. The catchment populations for two of the clinics (Naguru and Kiswa) are not permanent; people come and go. Apart from the highly mobile population, the people in these areas are also of different ethnic groups with different cultures and speaking different languages. Under these circumstances there is clearly little sense of local community and it is almost impossible to try to create one. The final clinic is the Kampala dispensary, located right in the centre of the city and which therefore does not have a catchment population which is locally residential.

Clearly, a different way of thinking about how to provide primary health care in these urban areas is needed. The Kampala experience so far has demonstrated how NGOs are often in an advantageous position not only to promote a primary health care approach in urban areas but also to perceive the limitations of the traditional approach in certain areas and to start working with local people to develop alternatives.

Khulna slum community health project
(Based on information from Quaji Ghiasuddin)

The problem of urban deprivation is growing in Bangladesh. Just over 20 per cent of the population, representing 23 million, live in towns. About half of these are in the four main cities of which Khulna is the third largest. The population of Khulna is more than one million and at least half are estimated to live on the borderline of starvation. Most of these people are legal slum dwellers who negotiate contracts with private landlords as opposed to squatters or pavement dwellers. The slums typically cover a small area, on average around a half acre, but the city has many such areas. The slums are growing rapidly from internal growth as much as migration in from rural areas.

Studies in 1989 reported that the infant mortality rate in poor urban areas was 180/1000 live births and the child mortality rate 114/1000. More than 60 per cent of children were malnourished and over ten per cent severely so. The main health problems reflect the poor living conditions: diarrhoeal diseases, tetanus and acute lower respiratory infections are the common causes of death while skin, eye and ear infections and worm infestations are widespread as are nutrient deficiencies of vitamin A and B2 (riboflavin).

Past and present government health policy and health service delivery structures have been developed for rural areas, as are the activities of nearly all NGOs working in health. SCF UK first worked in the Khulna district after the 1971 War of Liberation, providing emergency feeding for children. These activities soon developed into a network of basic curative health clinics, which were closed over the years as government services were established. From 1982, emphasis was given to preventative health work which included three small mother and child health clinics being opened in the slum areas of Khulna City.

In 1989, the project was reviewed and the objectives and plans rewritten. The main aim is to develop a low cost model community development project including a health component which could be copied by other agencies or the Government in other slum blocks of the city. The programme implementation strategies emphasize self-reliance, sustainability and active participation. The health component specifically aims to ensure access for the population, but particularly mothers and children, to basic health and other services or resources, such as clean water and credit.

The success of SCF UK's activities is reflected in health statistics in the slum areas of the programme. In 1992, three years into the project, the infant and child mortality rates in the SCF UK programme area had dropped to 54 and 75 respectively, compared with 72 and 88 in 1991. Almost half of the infant and child deaths occurred outside of the project area when families went to the rural areas for the harvest time. Of the other deaths, only one failed to get referred to a hospital in Khulna. Underlying these figures is probably the success achieved with the preventative integrated activities of the programme. Regular growth monitoring and action has ensured that only rarely does a child become severely malnourished. Coverage rates of immunization of children and women of reproductive age have been consistently maintained at 95 per cent or more over the last three years. Nearly all children receive vitamin A supplementation and almost all births are attended by a trained TBA. The use of family planning methods are started and continued by 80 per cent of couples in the areas where SCF UK first started working. Uptake has been slower elsewhere, as expected, but coverage is still over 60 per cent in the whole project area.

The SCF UK programme in Khulna City illustrates three aspects of how an NGO can contribute to health care in urban areas. The traditional strength of NGOs is exploited by working with urban communities. However, wider development goals for the city are addressed through a concern from the start with ensuring sustainability and with planning expansion into other slum areas.

The SCF UK programme in Khulna has highlighted a number of issues around working with urban communities: the appropriate scale for community units, ensuring that the community really wants the programme, the maintenance of communication between community workers and their communities and the time needed to build up a community based programme.

The SCF UK project operates on a small scale approach, not in terms of its potential overall coverage, but by dividing the potential coverage area into distinct geographical areas. Within the project, these areas cover about 600 households, with the same activities being carried out in each, although different areas will be at different stages in the implementation strategy. The small scale nature facilitates communication and understanding, and also access by the beneficiaries to SCF UK staff and *vice versa*. This approach aims to make each area's activities localized and thus to encourage the interest and involvement of the majority of the local population. The localized nature of the project is reflected in the personnel policies of SCF UK. The community workers must be young, literate women with children who live in the slums where they work. If they move out of the project area, then they lose their jobs. They are elected by their communities and are adequately, although not highly, paid.

Ensuring that a community really wants the project, is committed to the aims and feels involved fully is critical for community based activities to work. SCF UK has made community commitment a prerequisite for involvement in a new slum area. Work only starts in an area after the community has demonstrated their commitment by providing a simple building without charge within the target slum area, often a bamboo and thatch hut with a mud floor, with basic furniture and has agreed to cover all repair and running costs. No family is included in the programme unless it pays a registration fee of five taka in advance, and a flat fee of two taka is collected at the door from all clinic patients. This policy is applied across all SCF UK community based activities in the Khulna slums. For example, before SCF UK organizes to have a well installed through the local government, the total installation costs of tubewells are collected from slum dwellers and two women caretakers elected and trained from the community. As a result, there is a public demonstration of the contribution to and the ownership of the programme by both parties. Without this, a relief mentality would still probably prevail and the task of encouraging full involvement be very difficult. The full involvement from the start is essential to meet the long term aim of full ownership, control and payment of direct costs by the community.

The local population must view the community workers' services as theirs, not something different or special, therefore much attention has been given to ensuring that lines of communication are kept open and easy between beneficiaries and the community workers. Simple measures have been taken by community workers such as sitting with people rather than talking across a table or desk at them. Clinic waiting rooms are designed as open spaces rather than fenced-in lines or a row of benches. Uniforms are not worn by SCF UK staff. The activities of the project are integrated. Unlike the government services, which are delimited into categories such as immunization, family planning, curative health and so forth, all community health workers are trained to undertake all of the community based activities in their respective communities. The standard is basic (no doctor works in the programme in a medical role) but cheap and effective. The roles and work of the community workers and the network of community volunteers, mostly trained birth attendants, is easily understood by the community population. In this way, the community members effectively become monitors of the project activities.

The experience of building up a project which involves the slum dwellers themselves from the start took some years to establish good relations, understanding and mutual trust. From the outset, SCF UK's interest was in providing preventative health care. However, local people gave first priority to good curative services. Good relationships between the community and the NGO were built up by providing curative care for a few years to meet the local immediate demand and priorities. This in turn established a solid basis for introducing the aims of preventative care. Once preventative services were introduced, a further time period was necessary for the effects of preventative measures such as immunization, growth monitoring, family planning and health education to be evident to the community, valued and accepted. At this stage, local demand was seen to rise strongly.

Long term sustainability has been a central concern for the project design from the start. The project has concentrated on building on resources already available in the community and has reviewed the affordability of the components which would need to be covered by the community for the activities to continue. Lastly, mechanisms are being developed for handing over the management of health care to the community.

As far as possible, nothing is given or done by SCF UK which either reduces, replaces or prevents the community relying on its own abilities and resources. For instance, safe delivery kits are not given to either TBAs or prospective mothers but TBAs are advised to buy the necessary materials from local materials. Whether they pass the cost on to the mothers is their decision.

The costs of the project which the community has to meet for the work to continue with no SCF UK inputs must be affordable to the population. In 1992, these costs on average per month were 17.5 taka per family for all the project's activities (ie not just the health component). Together with other costs for salaries and related expenditure for community supervisors and SCF UK staff team leaders and with the overheads for staff and setting up the SCF UK office the monthly total was 47.5 taka. The affordability of the costs to be borne locally has been positively assessed through discussions with the slum dwellers and baseline surveys on family income and housing rents.

In each area, a community committee has been formed and meets monthly to discuss progress, problems and plans with the minutes posted publicly in community centres and bazaars. Rules for the formation of committees ensure priority goes to beneficiary women's representation, but also include community workers and volunteers and local landlords. Whilst the latter were suspicious of SCF UK's motives at first, the initial emphasis on popular and understandable work (curative care of sick children) could not be seen by them as a threat and thus reduced the likelihood of any interference and in fact resulted in a positive view of the project. Their inclusion in committees promotes openness and reduces suspicion and rumour. In addition to these committees, periodic workshops are held for groups of mothers from the slum areas and occasional general community meetings are held at the local primary schools. Again, minutes are taken and displayed publicly.

Results have been encouraging. Committees have developed from acting as the ears and mouths of the communities into being the agency initiating actions. The most important of these initiatives, now standard in all areas, is the establishment of community referral funds. One taka a month is collected from each registered slum family whenever the fund falls below a certain level, and used at the discretion of the committee to pay for the medical costs of patients referred to a hospital by the community workers. In a couple of instances, this community support initiative has gone even further and funds have been used to help families who have hit a particularly difficult phase economically, such as where a main income earner falls ill. Other committee initiatives have included the organization of common latrine cleaning rotas, regular rubbish clearance days and the improvement and maintenance of lanes and ditches in the area.

The strategy for spreading the model combines a mix of an additive approach where the activities of the NGO expand and a rolling approach where the NGO moves areas. The project started from the three original areas and slowly expanded to cover nine slums by the end of 1992, covering 17,000 people. The project plans to continue expansion to 12 areas. From that point onwards, the expansion will be made through a rolling process. New areas will be added as the activities in the established areas become largely independent of the NGO's inputs. The resources of the NGO can then be used to start up community activities in a new slum area.

The impact and benefits derived from the approach taken in the Khulna slums project have already been demonstrated at this stage. The next step in the project is to agree to a method to collect enough money to cover direct costs by the local populations. If this is possible, the communities will also need some training to become self-sufficient in their managerial as well as technical skills. At this stage, the role of the NGO will change. SCF UK will act purely as a background supporter, freely accessible as a source of information and advice, possibly acting as a banker and auditor, to a network of small slum organizations. This represents an innovative strategy for NGOs working with primary health care in urban areas both in the capacity building of networks of slum organizations and in the long term relationship planned between the NGO and the local urban communities.

SAVE THE CHILDREN – USA

(Based on information from Katherine Kaye)

Like most American NGOs working in international health and development, the American Save the Children (SC US) has based its programmes mainly in rural areas. However, with a mission of achieving lasting improvement in the lives of disadvantaged children, the international department now has three active urban projects involving health in Amman in Jordan, Manila in the Philippines and Jakarta in Indonesia. All of the international programmes are community based and rely upon community health workers. SC US has been working in Jakarta, Indonesia, for the last ten years, in partnership with the local health department. A review of the activities in Jakarta demonstrates two roles for an NGO in urban areas. First, the focus on community based actions and the partnership with the city level health department gives the NGO a bridging function between the two. Second, the NGO can carry out surveys and other assessments of primary health care activities at the local delivery level and identify modifications to improve their appropriateness in different urban settings.

Indonesia's pattern of urbanization resembles that seen elsewhere in the developing world. Between 1980 and 1985, the nation's annual urban growth rate was 5.5 per cent, more than five times that in rural areas. The proportion of Indonesians living in cities is expected to increase from 26 per cent at present to over 36 per cent by 1995, still resulting to a large degree from continued high rates of rural to urban migration. The level of urban poverty first exceeded that of rural poverty in 1981, and the incidence of poverty is declining more slowly in urban than in rural areas. According to the Indonesia Central Bureau of Statistics, 23 per cent of urban residents live in poverty. With a population of 7.9 million in 1985, Jakarta accounted for 19 per cent of the total Indonesia urban population. By the year 2000, Jakarta's population is expected to reach 15.7 million (Government of Indonesia/UNICEF 1989 Harpham et al 1988).

The government of Indonesia adopted a primary health care approach and established local health posts called posyandus, initially in rural areas. The posyandu aims to provide 'an integrated package of mother and child health, family planning, nutrition, immunization and diarrhoeal disease control into a service point at the village or hamlet level' (Leimana 1989). The posyandu activities are supported through the district health department (puskesmas) who provide personnel to deliver immunizations, prenatal care and family planning; establish monitoring systems for children attending the clinics; and train community health workers (volunteers called kaders) to conduct growth monitoring sessions, record immunization and growth monitoring data and to promote posyandu attendance. The Indonesian Government plans to increase the number of posyandus, particularly in the most populous provinces. The posyandu model has also been transposed into urban areas, particularly the poorer areas.

Support of posyandu activities was integral to the work of SC US in Jakarta starting from 1986 in just one slum area (Duri Utara). In 1989, this programme was expanded into the adjacent slum area of Duri Selatan and into nearby Jelambar Baru, bringing the total population covered by the project to 62,000. SC US health staff organized health planning workshops for community residents, helped the community health workers maintain a community based health information system, organized nutrition education sessions for mothers with malnourished children, involved some parents of malnourished children in income generating programs, distributed a larvicide to prevent dengue, and attempted to upgrade posyandu activities through better management and coordination with the puskesmas. These health activities were complemented by two much smaller projects initiated by the NGO to provide credit unions and day care centres.

In August 1991, SC US carried out a survey of 690 mothers and 593 children (aged younger than three years) who lived in the communities of Duri Utara and Jelambar Baru. At the time of this survey, SC US had been operating in Duri Utara slightly over five years and in Jelambar Baru less than one year. Interviewers who conducted the survey were either members of the NGO health team or community health workers. The study was designed in part to determine whether services offered through posyandus are accessed by the entire community or specific groups, and to measure the health impact of those services.

Among the conclusions generated by the survey were a number of points which have general application for primary health care activities in other urban settings.

1. Socio-economic heterogeneity often exists in even the poorest urban communities and should be considered in the design of programmes for health and health care. Like many urban slums, Duri Utara and Jelambar Baru are ethnically and economically heterogeneous. Although all population groups are of low income, the Chinese population tends to be relatively better off in both areas. The Chinese comprise 25 per cent of the population in both areas and ethnic Indonesians the remainder. Patterns of using health services differ according to socio-economic status. Wealthier residents tend to obtain primary health care from private providers, while local government clinics (posyandus and clinics based at subdistrict health departments) provide care for poorer residents. Health status in terms of malnutrition and diarrhoea prevalence was higher, as usually found, amongst the poorest groups. And yet preventative health practices, such as use of oral rehydration therapy and immunization coverage, were better among those routinely using government clinics. Although the higher socio-economic status of those who seek care from private providers may help counterbalance any of their poorer health practices, those not themselves practising preventative health care not only place themselves at greater risk, but also others.

2. Preventative approaches to primary health care need to decide how the government services will relate to the private providers found in urban areas. Urban primary health care activities need to consider

how to improve the preventative health care behaviours of those more affluent residents using private sources for health care. Since standards of preventative care in the for profit sector seem to be worse than those in the public sector, arguments that greater involvement of the private sector improves health care quality through competition need to be treated with caution (Bennett 1992). One approach for improving the protective health behaviours of more affluent residents could be accomplished by improving the standard of care offered by private providers, for example, through training programmes, increased regulation by the municipal health department and financial incentives. On the other hand, encouraging use of the posyandu by wealthier residents offers an opportunity to build greater community cohesion. This new population of posyandu users are more able to demand effective services at the local clinic, such as the monthly presence of an immunization team from the subdistrict health department. A third advantage for the public health services of encouraging use by wealthier residents is the potential for institutionalizing a system of a sliding fee scale which could be used to subsidize health services for the poorest members of the community. Thus, in some cities, NGOs may function most effectively by better equipping the public sector to meet current and potentially increasing demand.

3. The advantages and disadvantages for implementing a community based health information system in urban areas need to be considered against the benefits which the system is expected to bring to community residents and public and/or private health care providers. The proposed aims of a community based health information system (HIS) are to promote equity in use of health services and community empowerment.

   Promoting equity in health service use through a community based HIS operates by identifying and reaching out to groups who are often neglected. The achievement of this goal requires that all community residents be registered in the system.

   Completeness of HIS data was assessed through a household survey. The proportion of families who were unenrolled was 12 per cent in the community where SC US had operated longest and 18 per cent in the community where programme activities had started more recently. Those who had not been enrolled were more likely to be poor and recent migrants, high risk groups which proponents of community based information systems hope most to capture. Approximately 20 per cent of family migrations (either outmigrations or relocations within the project area) had not been recorded in the HIS records. Moreover, the two communities were considered to have a relatively low proportion of recent migrants for a poor slum area: fewer than 10 per cent of survey respondents had moved into the project area within the last two years and approximately 75 per cent had lived there longer than five years.

   Failure to maintain accurate records was related to three kinds of factors. Expansion of the programme without proportional staff increases led inevitably to reduced supervision. Political change following elections brought with it change in the appointments of the community health workers, which was decided by the local political administration. New community health workers then needed to be trained which disrupted the continual information collection. The SC US community based information system paralleled the government system based on clinic visits. The community health workers ended up spending a large proportion of their time updating the government records from the SC US system at the expense of making home visits for routine data collection.

The extent to which health benefits were associated with enrolment was unclear. Although enrolled mothers were more likely than unenrolled mothers to know and to use oral rehydration therapy, to have their 12 to 36 month old children fully immunized and to use family planning, these differences disappeared when economic status was controlled apart from that in immunization levels. The persistence of a difference in immunization status may therefore reflect an association between higher levels of government clinic use for immunization with enrolment into the information system amongst poor mothers.

Scarce resources and concerns about programme sustainability often lead to over-reliance upon volunteers to act as community health workers. A number of problems in using volunteers have emerged in urban areas. The urban poor may have much less time available for volunteer activities compared with their rural counterparts. The demands of a cash economy and the absence of traditional support from an extended family are likely to preclude participation of the poorest members of the community in volunteer activities thereby making it less likely that the poorest households will be visited. It is difficult to perceive how volunteers could visit homes frequently enough to maintain reliable information about vital events. Only intensive training can enable a volunteer community health worker to distinguish between such events as stillbirths and early neonatal deaths and to identify common causes of morbidity and mortality. Inevitably volunteer community health workers will have a high turnover with new training inputs constantly required. An NGO needs to consider whether at the end of the external inputs the responsibility and costs for training will be taken over by the local health authorities or a community organization.

Proponents of community based health information systems view them as tools to achieve community empowerment as well as greater equity. The argument is that as community residents learn to collect and interpret health data, they become better able to assess and address their own health needs. In this programme, however, overworked project health staff tended to emphasize the system's potential for generating vital events rates which could be used to monitor programme impact. While health information was occasionally channelled back into the community through meetings with community leaders, little attempt was made to determine either whether such forums truly represented all the diverse groups in the community (eg mothers, new migrants, Chinese residents, the very poor) or whether they increased community demand for services. There was also little effort on the part of health programme staff to work systematically with the community health workers or other community members to improve their ability to interpret health data.

At the end of the programme, however, there was evidence that some aspect of the SC US programme did in fact increase community awareness of the importance of primary and preventive health care. For example, community leaders supported the agency's efforts to create within the subdistrict health department a position which would provide supervisory support to the community health workers. Even more impressive was the willingness of these community leaders to designate part of their community endowment fund to pay the transportation expenses of such a supervisor in order to facilitate the ability to work with the community health workers in the field. A health information system which does succeed in raising local awareness about health and health needs will only be useful in redressing inequities in access to health if the local providers are able and willing to respond to increased demands. NGO health staff may need to work with public or private health care providers to improve the capacity and quality of their services.

The SC US Jakarta experience suggests that the establishment of an HIS which parallels the government system is counterproductive. Most costs of maintaining any HIS will eventually be borne by some level of government. Thus, NGO staff should understand the existing government recording system and assess health department interest in a community based approach. If the health department has already established a framework for a community based system, the NGO should work as much as possible within that framework, training existing government personnel as supervisors of community HIS workers and assisting in the achievement of greater efficiency.

4. Despite the concentration of tertiary care centres in cities, the urban poor in developing countries were generally thought to have little access to hospitals. Whatever access they did have was perceived as having no impact on overall community health (Harpham et al 1988). In the Jakarta communities, on the other hand, utilization of hospital services was higher than expected, at least for curative care. Delivery in hospital was common, especially among more affluent women, but even among poorer women the proportion of deliveries attended by traditional birth attendants was much lower than the 65 per cent observed nationally (Government of Indonesia/UNICEF 1989). Moreover, numbers of infant and child deaths in the two urban communities were lower than expected on the basis of national mortality rates, suggesting that in case of serious illness, access to hospitalization may avert death. Such access affects mortality rates and the overall spectrum of causes of mortality, and thus morbidity may be a better index than mortality of health conditions in slums.

However, access to hospital services may not be similar in all slums. Longer settlement of an area and greater stability of the population, as is the case in Duri Utara and Jelambar Baru, permits the evolution of greater community organization (Rifkin 1987) and may also change patterns of service utilization among the urban poor. In any given slum, patterns of hospital use should be clarified. An assumption that the urban poor will not seek care at hospitals should not preclude the possibility of working with a range of such institutions in cities to expand access to comprehensive health care, including curative as well as preventive services.

In the specific case of mother and child health services, the proximity of hospital based obstetric care offers a potential for early referral of complications which usually does not exist in rural areas. At the same time hospital delivery of uncomplicated births is not desirable especially where it severely strains limited facilities. Information about appropriate indications for seeking hospital care should be included in all urban prenatal care programs and arrangements should be made with hospital based providers to ensure availability of appropriate emergency services. On the community side, NGOs could work with credit unions or savings groups to develop insurance funds for hospitalization. Institution based personnel should also be acting to reverse the trend toward bottle feeding – which is observed most strikingly among wealthier women in these communities and who are those most likely to deliver in hospital. UNICEF's 'Baby-friendly hospital initiative' provides a model for this type of activity.

5. Children's nutritional status and incidence of diarrhoea demonstrated a close relationship between health and economic and environmental factors. The prevalence of malnutrition among all children is high: 44 per cent are mildly malnourished (weight for age between 75 per cent and 89 per cent of median); 22 per cent are moderately malnourished (between 60 per cent and 74 per cent of median); and 3 per cent are severely malnourished (less than 60 per cent of median). Levels of moderate and severe malnutrition were highest among children from the poorest families. The community wide incidence of diarrhoea was also high: 28 per cent of mothers reported at least one child under three with diarrhoea in the last month, and 7 per cent reported at least one under three year old hospitalized for diarrhoea in the last year. Diarrhoea was reported significantly more often by poorer mothers. Poorer families were also more likely to purchase water from vendors rather than to obtain it from an indoor tap or hydrant, and a trend towards higher incidence of diarrhoea among those who had to buy water persisted even after control for economic status.

The persistence of malnutrition among children who had taken part in an extensive growth monitoring programme shows that a selective intervention unaccompanied by adequate follow up is likely to fail. Follow up can only occur in the presence of a health infrastructure capable of delivering comprehensive care. Such infrastructure permits uninterrupted delivery of selective technologies and adequate follow up (with curative care, if necessary) of those identified as high risk (Rifkin and Walt 1986) By establishing local health clinics, the Indonesian government has taken an important step towards creating this type of infrastructure; now, to realize the potential of these clinics, it is necessary to strengthen delivery of preventive services at the posyandus and to institute on-site curative care or effective referral.

The clear association between health status, and economic and environmental factors indicates that even a comprehensive health care system needs to be part of a multisectoral approach. Nutritional rehabilitation of children detected as being severely malnourished during growth monitoring sessions does not address what is usually the root cause of the problem: absolute poverty. This case study offered some evidence, however, that increasing opportunities for income generation was by itself an inadequate solution. Children of poor mothers who were involved in income generating activities were more likely to be malnourished than were children of women who did not work for cash income. It will be important to make some form of child care accessible to working mothers. Further qualitative studies are needed to determine whether water sold by vendors is contaminated at the time of purchase or whether unsanitary conditions within households that must purchase water (the poorest in these communities) are more likely to be responsible for high rates of diarrhoea. If water is in fact contaminated at time of sale, the public health and sanitation departments could cooperate to develop a licensing system for vendors. The importance of cooperation between municipal health and water and sanitation departments is underscored. NGOs could perform a valuable service by facilitating such cooperation.

These lessons led to a greater awareness within the agency that uniquely urban development problems sometimes require approaches different from those used in rural areas. Following the survey, the organization modified its activities for strengthening primary health care in urban areas.

Health and development activities have been much more intensively concentrated on target groups. Save the Children's health programme in Jakarta now covers a population of approximately 14,000 in the four poorest neighbourhoods of Jelambar Baru. Target groups identified are new migrants, women factory workers, commercial sex workers, pregnant women and families in which one or more children are severely malnourished or delayed in their immunizations. At least 10 per cent of the households in these target areas are headed by women. The health information system has been simplified to reflect this sharper focus. Regular home visits are made only to members of targeted groups, communication between community health workers and commercial sex and factory workers, however, usually takes place in the setting of a health centre rather than in an individual home.

Community health workers are now expected to function more as case managers. In recognition of their dissatisfaction with a volunteer status long term, a revolving loan mechanism, the Kader Productivity Fund, has been established to provide some financial incentive for the performance of health promotion activities and the delivery of certain services such as nutritional rehabilitation of severely malnourished children.

Experience from the Child Survival programmes emphasized the need to institutionalize responsibility for the training and supervision of the community health workers. Consequently, SC US has encouraged the subdistrict health department to designate one of its clerical level workers as Health Coordinator, with responsibility for community workers recruitment and performance. The Health Coordinator Training Module which is being developed by SC US will be piloted in those subdistrict health departments which serve the NGO's programme area. If the Health Coordinators prove to be effective, the module can be used more widely to train this level of government health worker. The willingness of local political leaders to allocate a portion of their community savings to cover transportation costs for the Health Coordinator suggests a higher community priority given to primary health care needs and may herald greater cooperation between health department and community.

CONCLUSION

The examples presented from Kampala, Khulna and Jakarta all demonstrate how the traditional strength of NGOs in working at the local level with people to promote their health is particularly critical in urban areas at this time. The realization that the expanding urban populations are inadequately served by hospital oriented health care systems in cities has been accompanied by many initiatives to develop an urban primary health care approach, local urban district health systems and so forth.

The extensive experience of NGOs in primary health care in rural areas makes them ideal agencies to establish a link between communities and city health departments. Strategies for working with urban communities may follow similar lines as in rural areas. It is important to note, however, the Khulna experience which highlighted the time scale necessary to build up truly community based health activities in urban areas. In Kampala, clearly defined or coherent communities did not exist in many areas of the city. In these areas, a different kind of approach is needed.

The problem typically faced by NGOs active in development is how to scale up their impact. Three strategies are demonstrated in the examples. In Uganda, activities were focused on building rehabilitation and mother and child health, at least initially. By concentrating on key services, the NGO was able to work in all the public health clinics in the city, both at clinic and at community level. In Jakarta, the first phase of activities involved an additive approach to expansion. After reviewing the successes and constraints, the NGO has similarly focused its activities to increase impact. In this case, however, the focus is on population groups rather than health services as such. Perhaps the most innovative approach was seen in Khulna. The project aimed to develop a local model which could in theory be expanded indefinitely if funds were available, following a sort of building block approach. The emphasis on sustainability from the start in fact will allow the NGO to stop work in one district and move its resources to a new one in the future.

As cities continue to expand, health policy makers and city planners need a better understanding of the way people are living their lives in urban areas and the implications for health and health care delivery. NGOs, with a local level focus and the flexibility to be innovative, should be major actors in exploring, initiating and evaluating new models.

REFERENCES

Bennett, S (1992) Promoting the Private Sector: A Review of Developing Country Trends *Health Policy and Planning*, vol 7 no 2 pp97–110

Clark, J Z (1990) *Democratizing Development: The Role of Voluntary Organizations* Kumarian Press, West Hartford, Connecticut

Edwards, M and Hulme, D (1992) *Making a Difference* Earthscan, London

Government of Indonesia/UNICEF (1989) *Situation Analysis of Children and Women in Indonesia*

Harpham, T Lusty, T and Vaughan, P (1988) *In the Shadow of the City: Community Health and the Urban Poor*, Oxford University Press, Oxford

Leimana, S (1989) Posyandu: A Community Based Vehicle to Improve Child Survival and Development *Asia-Pacific Journal of Public Health* vol 3 no 4 pp264–267

Rifkin, S (1987) Primary Health Care, Community Participation and the Urban Poor: A Review of the Problems and Solutions *Asia-Pacific Journal of Public Health* vol 1 no 2 pp57–63

Rifkin, S and Walt, G (1986) Why Health Improves: Defining the Issues Concerning 'Comprehensive Primary Health Care' and 'Selective Primary Health Care' *Social Science & Medicine* vol 23 no 6 pp559–566

Save the Children Fund UK (1992) *Statement on Health Sector Policy in the Overseas Department* February, London

ACKNOWLEDGEMENTS

Many thanks go to the two NGOs for providing information on their activities. Peter Poore provided time and information to discuss SCF UK's approach to health and urban health. Mike O'Dwyer coordinated the collection of information on SCF UK activities in Uganda from the field staff there. Katherine Kaye was supported by the SC US staff in Indonesia – (Mike and Estela Novell), by colleagues working with urban health issues in the Philippines – (Susan Dawson and David Claussenius); in Jordan – (Maha Shadeed); and Colombia – (Monica Ortega); and by colleagues at the head office in Westport – (Warren Berggren). Sarah Atkinson previously worked on the Urban Health Programme at the London School of Hygiene and Tropical Medicine, funded by the Overseas Development Administration, UK.

13

View from the Slums of Asia – the Experience of a Christian Missionary Group

Michael Duncan and Christian Auer

INTRODUCTION

Servants is a Christian missionary movement that has various ministries among the urban poor of Asia. It is a basic tenet of the organization that its workers live in the slums, and from this base seek to involve themselves in the life of the community. Through this kind of contact, needs can be gradually discerned, and ministries come into being in cooperation with the people themselves. The organization does not concentrate on one kind of project, but attempts a holistic approach to the problems of the slum dwellers. 'Development' is seen not only in terms of practical activities like income generation schemes, community development, emergency relief (eg help with hospital bills, reconstruction after fires, funeral expenses), but also less concrete ones, like supporting the efforts of local churches to work towards equality and justice.

Many needs are connected with health, and Servants has become involved in projects like establishing clinics, providing credit facilities for the purchase of medicines, programmes for immunization, help with family planning, and educational aspects like health seminars and a 'child to child' health education scheme. Servants works together with local organizations such as churches, and with other NGOs.

This chapter is limited to the area of health care, and draws mainly on the organization's experience in Manila in the Philippines. It does not try to assess the performance of the various health care services provided, but rather explores some of the concepts that are important for Servants, and influence the way its members work. The role often played by medical practitioners – as people who come from outside the community and tend to offer 'top down', specialized and professional services – is considered in some detail, and alternative, more relational and holistic ways of approaching the problem of extending effective health care in poor urban areas are discussed.

THE SERVANTS MOVEMENT AND ITS AIMS

The organization was founded in 1980, when a group of New Zealand Christians met to discuss how best their small country could play a part in transforming the slums of Asia. For this group, there was no artificial division between the spiritual and the physical; nor did they think that the former was more important than the latter. Their concern was for the whole person and his or her quality of life in the widest sense.

The experience of the organization over the last ten years has encouraged its workers to see spiritual ministries and other ministries, like health care, as partners that go hand in hand. Health is closely linked with economic, environmental, emotional and spiritual factors. Often, renewal has to happen *inside* the people before physical, health and social needs can be addressed. For example, it is difficult to treat a person for tuberculosis if he or she is entrapped in drug abuse, alcoholism and criminality. One of the most important processes is the attempt to understand the underlying problems in a situation, such as corruption. This discussion can lead both expatriates and local people to a reassessment of the situation and of what needs to be done.

The aim of Servants is not to provide solutions from outside but to *empower* the poor, ie to help them to detect, develop and apply their own resources and abilities. It is vital that the work be *resource based* and not *deficiency based*. There is a danger of seeing only the problems and deficiencies in a community. This approach does not enhance community participation and development.

The organization now includes people from several different cities: Manila (17 expatriate staff; start 1983), Bangkok (eight; 1987), Dhaka (two; 1990), Phnomh Penh (ten; 1993). The Servants teams work closely with national groups, with the ultimate aim that they will take over what has been started by expatriates.

Servants is financed by the home churches and friends of the missionaries. In 1992, in the Philippines, Servants spent US $184,000 on ministries among the poor: 22 per cent for education (mainly preschools and supporting children and young adults in their education), 21 per cent for emergency relief among people affected by the eruption of Mount Pinatubo, 18 per cent for income-generating projects, 14 per cent for community projects (eg water and electric power supply), and 5 per cent for health care. The remaining 20 per cent was used for supporting Christian churches in poor urban areas and for helping people who had suffered from outbreaks of fire, and for other ministries.

In the same year, the living expenses of the 16 expatriates (including nine children), the rent of an office and of a retreat house, the salary of the secretary in the office, and maintenance, amounted to about US$100,000. Of the money given for projects, only 3 per cent was deducted for administrative expenditure related to the projects. In looking at the figures, it is also important not to forget that there are many important activitites which require a great deal of staff time and energy but tend not to appear in project balance sheets. These include counselling and a lot of informal health education.

Table 13.1 *The four phases of the ministry of Servants in poor urban communities in Manila*

Phase	Main features & time	Activities/approach	Lessons learnt
I 1983–1987	Adjustment to slum life Acceptance into community	Move into slum Listen to the people Share daily struggles (eg power and water shortages)	The slum inhabitants have much to offer and teach First world medicine and practice often divorced from slum life The slum inhabitants are alienated by outside professionals
II 1987–1989	Work *for* the poor	Dole out Focus on curative medicine Top down; we are the professionals	Dependency created Dole out and top down enhances the slum inhabitant's sense of weakness and creates new power structures under the control of benefactor Does not effect long term changes or address the reasons for ill health Money does not solve everything Sickness not only physical but also social and spiritual
III 1989–1992	Evaluate the past Work *with* the people	Consult with the people Community development Preventitive health care	The slum inhabitants want to participate They have many skills in community development and health Preventive healthcare not sufficient in itself (curative also needed)
IV 1992 on-wards	Integration of above into holistic model of healthcare and mission	Community health focus Integration of spiritual and physical Clinics with partial payments for medicines Cooperative drug stores that are community based and initiated Networking with other agencies	Approach used in healthcare dependent on stated needs of community Timing of approach also important

THE RATIONALE FOR LIVING IN THE SLUMS

A big difference between Servants and most other organizations – both governmental and Non-governmental – is that the Servants workers actually live in the slums among the most disadvantaged people. The rationale behind this is not only theological. The members of the team do not want to be perceived by the community as 'outsiders'. They are fully aware that even when they live in the community, people from more prosperous circumstances cannot fully *identify* with the poor. However, they can *participate* in the life of the community, even to the point of entering into some of the people's struggles, and suffering from some of the same problems.

When the Servants team began work in the slums, they found that people in deprived urban areas had been growing more and more disenchanted with the professionals and the experts coming into their communities on a 'nine o'clock to five o'clock' basis. They asked how the doctors could possibly treat and cure their complaints if they did not know them and their physical environment, or understand their 'culture of poverty' (Lewis 1966).

After living in an area for some time, the Servants workers became aware that health care was more acceptable when those who provided it were 'insiders', who lived with the people, and were prepared to learn from them, listen to them and understand them. Insiders do not come only to provide something, but also to receive. The process of providing health care – or in a wider sense the restorative process – is more effective when it takes place in a context of relational and compassionate solidarity with the sick and the disadvantaged.

Most professionals working with the poor in Asia live in first world suburbs in third world cities. From the comfort of their air-conditioned houses they go to the slums and do their work, only to retreat again later in the day. This approach only serves to underline to the poor that yet again they are seen as objects to be treated. This 'subject/object' division is one of the reasons for the growing disenchantment of the poor with Western medicine. Western medicine often reduces the sick person to being an object to be treated. It is the doctor who is the subject, the 'healing agent', and not the patient.

Health professionals who actually live in the community can communicate a different dynamic in providing health care. Activities aimed at restoring health become a joint or communal affair. The Servants workers found that if they themselves fell sick, it did not hamper their attempts to provide health care by making them less credible, but that on the contrary, it helped people to believe that they would really be understood, and trust began to develop. The development of trust and friendship in its turn influences people's health seeking behaviour; health care is likely to be more acceptable when it comes through someone who is perceived as being a member of the community.

This is well illustrated by the development of family planning in a small squatter community called Potrero. Many mothers living in conditions of poverty want to practise family planning, but financial and other constraints often hinder them (University of the Philippines 1987).

A woman working with Servants settled in Potrero, and became friendly with a mother with four children, who worshipped in the same small local church. Once trust had developed between them, the mother asked the Servants worker for advice about family planning, and the Servants worker helped her to make contact with a small Christian hospital which offers tubal ligation at a subsidized price. The operation was successful, and encouraged a friend of the first mother's, and subsequently other women, to undergo the operation. Most of these women are prepared not only to encourage others, but also to accompany them to the hospital.

When workers are actually living in the slums, and are trusted by the community, their example can also lead to a kind of informal health education that is much more effective than words. For instance, people who had watched how the Servants workers had treated their own sick children were much more easily convinced that a particular form of treatment – such as the frequent bathing of children with chickenpox – was appropriate, and to practise it themselves.

Learning is, however, a two-way process. A health worker who is part of the community will encounter folk medical practices, some of which may prove to be better and more appropriate than what 'Western' medicine has to offer. One of the Servants' workers describes such an encounter:

> *One day a mother came to the door of one of our families with a very distraught boy in tow. He was suffering from bad burns. We dressed them twice with very expensive medicines, but this did not prove effective. The mother then tried placing guava* (Psidium guajava) *leaves on the burns and they subsequently healed very rapidly. Perhaps we should have sought for local measures first.*

The Servants workers consider that their task is to seek out and work with what already exists, as well as to introduce some things from the outside that the people themselves cannot provide. This can be done most effectively by people who are trusted members of the local community. But it must be 'both... and', not 'either... or'.

SERVANTS' WORK IN MANILA

The work of the Servants organization in Manila can be divided into four phases (see Table 13.1). The initial phase was mainly one of coming to terms with what it actually meant to live in the slums as Western individuals or families, and attempting to become insiders in the community. In the second phase, the team began to do things for the poor. The third phase was a difficult one. Members of the community began to criticize the work, which led to an extremely painful process of reassessment, when the members of the team began to realize that they were still doing things for the poor rather than with them. The current phase is an attempt to bring together the insights from these three phases into a more integrated and holistic model for communal health development in poor urban areas.

Phase I: *moving into the slums*

It is not a simple matter for an individual or a family from a different culture and a different situation to move into a slum area to live. Over the years, the organization has developed a number of criteria on which to base the selection of a suitable place.

Firstly, the community has to be considered carefully. When a Westerner settles into a community, there is a danger that he or she may become too central, too noticeable. The bigger the slum, the more this problem is minimized – though it can never be eradicated. It is also important that the area should be one in which land tenure is secure enough for the Servants worker to be sure of being able to stay for some years. It may easily take two years for a worker to be 'adopted' by a community.

The community must be in need of an NGO working in its midst, and the Barangay Council (local political council) of the community must agree to a Servants worker moving into the area. The organization does not move into areas where its activities would compete with those of local churches, unless the team can usefully offer them support by bringing together representatives of the different churches to form a 'core group' to facilitate development in the community.

The situation must also be considered from the point of view of the Servants workers, if they are to remain long enough to become really integrated into the community and carry out an effective ministry. For families, it is better if the community is a 'slum of hope', where the degree of poverty is not so extreme, and vice and criminality are not too frequent. Questions like the availablility of schools are also important. Single people may move into a 'slum of despair', where poverty is even more acute and the prevalence of vice and crime are higher. The community should not be too far away from the Servants' retreat centre where the team meets regularly. Servants workers join Servants with two commitments: one, to the urban poor and the other, to the team.

Phase II: *the first experience*

In this phase, the Servants team members did a lot for the people in their slum area. The emphasis was on curative medicine and providing free drugs. A member of the team describes the experience of this phase thus:

> *Living in the slums day and night created a deep sense of shock. For many of us, this was our first real exposure to actual poverty. It was quite different from the "textbook poverty" that we had read about in the comfort of our living rooms back in New Zealand or elsewhere. Although we noted that the poor have resources and abilities, the deficiencies and urgent needs around us made a stronger impact on our hearts and minds. We became deficiency oriented, and our response was to create all manner of "dole out" mercy ministries. We thus became very much like other aid organizations, motivated by compassion and in need of money, medicines and organization. It was very much our "curing the poor". We, the professionals and experts, had come into the slums in order to do a lot for the people. This had two results. First, it*

created a spirit of dependency among the sick. Second, it inhibited community health. Individuals were being made whole, but the community was left untouched.

Phase III: evaluation and readjustment

The third phase began with apparent failure. The people of the community actually asked the Servants team to stop its mercy ministries. They argued that much of what the organization was doing for them was in fact damaging relationships and leading to communal breakdown. In other words, the social effect of all the programmes was actually proving harmful. The organization's 'individualistic' approach to health care, in choosing one person over another, was creating jealousy and misunderstandings. Its 'top down' approach was alienating the poor, who did not feel that they were playing an active part in the provision of health care in the community. They were simply beneficiaries of the process, not managers of the process, and they had little to do with its implementation. They felt demeaned by this. The team realized that in healing some part of the body they were causing a sickness of the spirit. Holistic health care was not being provided.

The team proceeded to analyse their original approach to health and health care in the slums, and came to the following conclusions:

1. When the team came into the slums with medical practitioners, medicines and money, the poor were attracted to these. The starting point in this health care delivery moved away from the people. It focused on the Western medical practitioner, who defined, assessed and reacted to the health problems of the people from his or her perspective.
2. In basing health and health care on what the organization had to offer, the team communicated to the poor – albeit unintentionally – that, 'What they had did not count for much in our scheme of things.' Not only had this dealt another blow to their already fragile self-esteem, but it had also reinforced in their minds the idea that foreign was superior, and local inferior.
3. The medical practitioners had become the élite of the slum; the patrons; the upper class of the community. Through being the providers they were elevated to the status of benefactors. The local people inevitably became the beneficiaries, reduced to being just patients.

One of the team describes the process of reassessment and evaluation thus:

> *Our money made it possible immediately to do much for the sick. We were so swept along by what our Western money could do that we ignored the sick people themselves. The sick began to disappear behind the piles of aid funds. All of this was unintentional, and at first we did not notice it. We just had not spent the necessary time simply sitting with the sick so as to get an insider's view, and learning to understand the health related issues that existed in the*

community, and how the people perceived these issues. We had not considered carefully what approaches there were to choose from, which were the most appropriate, and what might be the consequences of our choice. We had not taken time to discover the worldview and values of the people we were working among. Instead, as health professionals, we communicated the primacy of physical well-being, and the view that Western medicine was the way to this state of health. Medicine became the ultimate answer. But when this expectation was firmly in place, many people discovered that they could not afford the medicines. What was promised could not be delivered. The poor thus became victims of a gap between promise and fulfillment.

The situation not only produced problems for the community, but also put too great a strain on the team members: 'We became tired servants. We had become the focus; the providers; the "healers"; the experts. It was too great a strain to be all those things. We could not cope with not being able to help everybody. No one is meant to play God.'

Phase IV: new approaches

Having taken stock, and realized the consequences of their approaches in phase two, the Servants workers began to engage themselves more in community development and preventive health care. It was a shift away from 'one to one' relief projects towards projects that would benefit the whole community. Before a new programme was started, the members of the community were asked to discuss it amongst themselves. They had to own it, or ultimately it would not usher in sustainable community health.

The next section discusses some of the health projects carried out, their evolution over time and the lessons learned from them.

SERVANTS' EXPERIENCE

The clinic in Bagong Silang

Bagong Silang is a relocation area (also called resettlement area) in the periphery of Metro Manila. It has about 200,000 inhabitants, most of whom are poor or very poor. In June 1988 a nurse working with Servants went to live there. He was shocked by the high mortality (mainly due to diarrhoea, pneumonia and malnutrition) and morbidity (mainly due to diarrhoea, respiratory tract infections, skin infections, accidents and burns) around him, and the grossly insufficient existing health services. Therefore he started a clinic, after having asked the medical officer of the governmental health centre responsible for the area for permission. The approach was a purely curative one, including the distribution of free drugs where necessary, but there was also an immunization service offered once a month.

As time went on, and Servants workers got to know the health care system in Manila better, they encountered a number of factors that, they felt, added to the difficulties of promoting health. One doctor felt strongly that many of the doctors working in the city had been trained in a medical system which scarcely took into account that illness is more than a set of symptoms. The sick person was seldom educated so that disease would be less likely to occur in the future and the patient would feel confident enough to deal with the illness on his or her own the next time. Most patients – especially the poor – were kept dependent and ignorant. Furthermore, the omnipresent mass media and other carriers of promotion constantly praise all sorts of medicines (eg antidiarrhoeals, cough syrups, expensive multivitamins), causing the people and also some doctors to believe that drugs are needed for every illness.

In 1990, a medical doctor from New Zealand took over the clinic. Gradually, the approach began to include health education. Care was taken to explain their health problems to the patients, and to encourage good health behaviour. Handouts in the local language about the most common diseases were available to give to the patients. The patients had to give a symbolic financial contribution (five to ten pesos) for medicine. In 1991 and 1992 more than 1000 patients were seen each year.

Four women health volunteers were trained in basic health care, and became very committed to the clinic. As sincere Christian believers, they wanted to live out their faith by caring for others. Although they were poor themselves, they received no remuneration. Their role gradually changed as they became more experienced; in 1992, they began to make the diagnoses, give explanations and administer medicine. By 1993, they were working as a team with a Swiss nurse, and contributing their own knowledge of herbal medicine and their own insights into the problems of the patients. The Swiss nurse wrote: 'We enjoy working together. They ask questions, express doubts or otherwise supplement my suggestions about treatment, and I do well to take them seriously, because they often have a much better feeling for the situation than I do. It is a situation of mutual learning.'

At the end of 1992 this medical ministry of Servants in Bagong Silang became part of the health care ministry of a coalition of a number of different Christian NGOs. The four volunteers have moved on to start a drug cooperative in the area, under the auspices of SANGKOP, a network of Christian NGOs in Manila. This organization has developed a model for drug cooperatives which has worked successfully in other areas of Manila and which could be extended to the whole of the Philippines (see Boxes 13.1 and 13.2). The four volunteers went to seminars run by SANGKOP, to learn how to set up a drug cooperative in their own area. The first step was to carry out a survey to look at the most urgent health needs of their area. When they had confirmed that better access to lower priced medicaments was indeed a pressing need, they began the process of planning and setting up the cooperative.

The drug cooperative started with 78 member families, and by the beginning of 1994 there were 238. In addition, the cooperative has been able to provide a loan of US $110 to establish a second cooperative, with 90–100 member families, in another area of Bagong Silang.

Child to child health clubs

Because she felt that children were more open to new ideas than their elders, a doctor working with Servants, together with two mothers from the squatter area where she lived, started to teach children basic health care: for example, the importance of personal and environmental cleanliness, nutritious food, immunizations and very basic care for the sick. The aim was not that the children should become the health care providers in their households, but that they should be able to help their mothers and brothers and sisters, and even assist others in the community.

'Health clubs' were set up, with groups of 10–15 children aged nine to 12 years, who were given a basic eight week health course. Nearly half of the first 42 children who finished a course are still obviously active: they meet regularly and do various things like cleaning in their communities.

In general, the effect of these health clubs has been encouraging; health prevention and promotion does take place and behavioural changes occur. However, their effectiveness depends on finding enough teachers – people with a good knowledge about basic health care and a gift for working with children. In the slums it is not easy to find people who are both capable and available. For 1994 it is planned to integrate the approach of child to child health clubs into the four existing preschools run by Servants.

Feeding programme in Kaingin Bukid

Kaingin Bukid is a squatter area in Metro Manila with roughly 800 families. There is a nearby government health centre, where residents have been trained to become Barangay (local district) Health Volunteers. However, these trained volunteers are generally not active. For the last two years there has been almost no involvement of NGOs in this community, apart from churches with spiritual ministries.

From July 1991 to May 1992, Servants operated a feeding programme. Fifty children (one to five years old) were given a nutritious meal five times a week. The meals were cooked by five mothers, residents of Kaingin Bukid, who received a remuneration of 500 pesos (= US$20) per month. One of the mothers was a nutritionist at the nearby government health centre. The object of this feeding programme was to feed malnourished children and also to educate their mothers. With this in mind it was planned to conduct a seminar once a month for *all* the mothers of the children enrolled in the scheme.

In May 1992, an evaluation was performed by a medical doctor in the Servants team. This revealed several deficiencies:

1. Five of the 50 enrolled children had normal weight when admitted to the feeding programme, in spite of the fact that a Servants worker had thoroughly explained to the local nutritionist that only malnourished children were to be accepted.
2. The cooked meals were nutritious and well prepared, but the mothers of the enrolled children were not involved in helping with the cooking, so a natural opportunity to share knowledge of what is

Box 13.1

A COMMUNITY BASED DRUGSTORE COOPERATIVE: THE SMOKEY MOUNTAIN EXPERIENCE

Maria Emma D Palazo, Manila, Philippines

The Community Drug Insurance Programme (CDIP) was set up by a Christian NGO, Tanging Binhi ng Buhay Foundation (The Seed of Life Foundation) and a people's organization in Smokey Mountain (SMBK – Association of Workers of Seeds in Health) in Manila, the Philippines.

In 1989 a survey by the Barangay Health Workers (BHWs: a Barangay is the smallest political unit) showed that there were about 10,000 people living on Smokey Mountain, an area of reclaimed land where garbage is dumped. An average family earned P800–1000 per month, mainly from scavenging. Patients attending the health centre generally had to buy prescribed drugs in shops at high prices.

Project Goals: To enable the residents to buy essential drugs at an affordable price, to educate the people about the importance of saving for their health needs, and to train BHWs in the proper handling and dispensing of drugs.

Seed money: In 1990, local organizations obtained a stock of drugs for the clinic as donations from drug companies, NGOs and the government. These drugs were supplied to patients at the clinic, who were asked to make a small cash contribution. A sum of P12,046 was thus obtained.

Informing the community: Before the drugstore was opened the community was thoroughly informed by BHWs visiting every house, and by the holding of community assemblies.

Implementation: The project started in 1990. Monthly contributions were P10 per month for families earning less than P1000 per month, and P25 for those earning more. These contributions formed the revolving fund for the cooperative. Members were given a 50 per cent discount on medicines. Non-members paid the full price plus a small profit for administrative expenses. BHWs took turns to look after the drugstore; two of them were trained in the bookkeeping required. They are paid an allowance of P500 per month by an NGO. Their work in the drugstore was overseen by a doctor and a midwife from the clinic. Drugs were mainly bought direct from generic drug companies who gave discounts for bulk orders.

Subsequent history: Since 1992 the BHWs and the SMBK have managed the CDIP by themselves; the doctor only oversees the accounts. Discounts on medicines have been reduced to 15 per cent from 50 per cent because the number of members has decreased. In 1994 the CDIP in Smokey Mountain had savings of US$1000 in the bank. The programme is being sustained by the daily drug sales and the membership fees.

Results: The project gave the people the opportunity of collectively sharing 1 per cent of their monthly earnings so that essential drugs could be available in the community at an affordable price. The CDIP won the Golden Award in a Health and Management Information System contest sponsored by the Philippine Department of Health and the German Government. It has become a model for setting up community drugstores in other parts of Manila and the Philippines (see Box 13.2).

Box 13.2

COMMUNITY DRUG INSURANCE PROGRAMME IN THE PHILIPPINES

Maria Emma D Palazo, Manila, Philippines

The original programme in Smokey Mountain was still continuing in 1994, with the BHWs managing the activities. The seed capital had reached $1000.

Expansion of the programme
Training workshops have been organized since 1992 for volunteer health workers from both urban and rural areas. By 1994, SMBK had trained 459 health workers from 190 barangays in 2–3 day training courses, followed by 6 months of monitoring and follow-up training.

Surveys
In the courses, health workers learn how to assess the health needs of the community by conducting a survey. The results will determine whether the people need a community managed drugstore and are willing to set one up.

Replication
By 1994, the SMBK had established 56 CDIPs (16 of them in Metro Manila). The goal is to establish CDIPs in 500 poor urban and rural communities within one year. In addition, the government plans to establish a further 1000. The capital for a cooperative comes from fund raising activities by the local people and from the monthly contribution of about 5 to 10 pesos (= 0.2 to 0.4 US$) per member family. The benefits that the members get are easy access to essential and commonly used drugs and a discount on the drugs purchased.

Basic principles
The CDIPs of SMBK have several important features designed to ensure the sustainability of the programmes even if NGOs or the government are no longer involved. These are:
• The CDIP should be a felt need of the community.
• The seed capital should come from the community.
• The families are encouraged to save 1 per cent of their income for health needs.
• The people of the community should manage the programme.

---

nutritious food was completely missed.
3. Enrolled children who failed to turn up at the feeding centre were not followed up.
4. The parents were not given their children's growth charts.
5. The monthly weighing was not done from November 1991 to March 1992.
6. Only three seminars were conducted, and not all mothers attended. The three seminars were performed in lecture style, which is not an effective health education method. There was, however, time for questions at the end of the seminars.

The following lessons were learned:

1. Firm guidelines and regular monitoring are essential.
2. The responsibilities of the staff involved in a programme need to be very clear.
3. Before a programme starts, those responsible need to find out about the knowledge and attitudes of the staff, and about the time they have available. In this feeding programme there was a misconception about the abilities and/or available time of the local nutritionist and the local supervisor.

A NEW PROJECT IN CAMBODIA

The delivery of health care is not a matter of choosing between alternatives – mercy ministries or community development; learning from the health professional or learning from the sick; working for the poor or with the poor; curative or preventive health care. Room must be made for all of these aspects, and each has its own particular contribution to make. However, decisions do have to be made about the sequence, and which activity should be emphasized at a particular time. Choices will depend on the context of the community, and should be directed by a study of its needs and resources, which cannot be done from a distance but must be done in the community, in collaboration with the people themselves.

The question of the choice of priorities is clearly illustrated by the work which Servants has now taken up in Cambodia. Here, in a country that has been ravaged by war for more than 20 years, there is a high morbidity and the existing health services are not sufficient. In such a situation, curative health care has to be high on the agenda, and so far the Servants team has been largely involved in improving existing health services.

The Servants team began work in Phnom Penh after detailed discussions with other NGOs, and also officials from the Ministry of Health and the municipal government. The organization still maintains close links with governmental agencies and NGOs. In March 1993, Servants received final approval from the Cambodian Government to start a health care project in Srok Mean Chey, one of the poorest areas of Phnom Penh. The team includes a number of experienced people, two of whom have worked in the Khmer refugee camps in the Thai-Cambodian border area.

The team members began by spending a considerable time on language study, and have now moved to slum areas of Phnom Penh to live. The work is at present concentrated on the small district hospital in Srok Mean Chey, where the members of the team work alongside the staff members, offering on the job training and support. The team has also been involved in helping with more formal educational projects, such as workshops on diarrhoea and vaccination. However, the Servants team hopes eventually to be able to concentrate on district based work, including preventive health care. Links will be maintained with the community of Srok Mean Chey, to ensure that the programme is community based and community relevant. Randomly selected members of the community will be asked about how they perceive the health services rendered. Health surveys will be conducted once a year to determine changes in the health status of the population, and the impact of the offered health services. The first survey was performed in September 1993.

In considering how to achieve the goal of improving the hospital services, the Servants team was confronted with the dilemma which faces many organizations; whether to support the current government system, in spite of its weaknesses, or whether to use resources from outside to achieve higher levels of care immediately. For example, it would have been possible to pay the Cambodian staff higher salaries, to increase motivation and enable them to work longer hours. This might have been successful in the short term, but would not have offered a sustainable improvement. Finally, Servants decided to work within the system as far as the day to day running of the hospital was concerned. However, realizing that the staff cannot live on their basic salaries alone, Servants has introduced a policy of remunerating staff for additional work, such as monthly vaccination 'outreaches'.

DEFICIENCY ORIENTED OR RESOURCE ORIENTED PROJECTS?

As they considered what had gone wrong in the second phase of their work, the Servants team members finally took to heart what they had already noticed while in phase one, namely that the members of the community were able to contribute a lot. They learned that

> *The slums are not just places of death. They are not all negative, full of misery, needs and deficiencies. Seeing them as negative encouraged us to "dole out" every imaginable medical aid. Now, however, we are learning to see these places positively, and that there are many resources and abilities available. It is our job to seek these out and work with them, as well as to introduce some things from the outside that the people themselves cannot provide.*

It is easy for organizations to become deficiency oriented rather than resource oriented. This tendency can even be encouraged by surveys designed to assess the needs of poor communities (McKnight 1989). Surveys are often an essential tool, but questionnaires have to be carefully designed not only to show the difficulties and problems, but to bring to light the resources and positive practices of the people involved. A well planned survey should help the people who are interviewed to see that they have resources and potential, and not only make them more aware of needs and deficiencies. Such a survey can be a basis for developing projects *with* the poor rather than *for* the poor – as was shown by the development of the drug cooperatives in Bagong Silang described in Boxes 13.1 and 13.2.

THE WORK OF THE HEALTH PROFESSIONAL AMONG THE POOR

The members of the Servants team found that the holistic approach to health care was not easy. They had to change in many ways, and this required courage. One of them writes:

> *There lies the problem of the professional. Most experts, medical doctors and the like, have imbibed the spirit of reductionism and specialization. Specialists tend to limit themselves to the particular practice, dogma and tradition of their own training. They have allowed their training to sum up their mode of operating, failing to recognize that this training, even though valid, is only a part of the whole. The challenge for the professional, therefore, is to stop limiting himself or herself to what he or she has done or been. Often, the specialist comes to the poor, identifies the deficiencies that he can address with his special training, and starts to work straight away, compelled or guided by the immediate need and his specialized knowledge. A resource oriented person, not limiting himself or herself by his or her specialization, could develop a ministry that would be based on the abilities of the poor and rooted in the community. Such a ministry would empower the people.*

The Servants' attempt to put an integrated model into practice underlined afresh that if medical workers are to remain committed to this demanding type of work for a long time it is essential for them to be part not only of the local community, but also of a supportive community of colleagues. Solitary workers often leave their engagement in poor communities after a short time because of burnout or disillusionment. It is important for the Servants workers that all the members of the team – medical and nonmedical – come together on a regular basis for times of refreshment and reflection.

An approach thus rooted in the community does not allow people to keep to their specializations. The members of the community come to the medical workers as whole persons, requesting that they also be whole people, so that together they can engage in the healing process. In this sense, a specialist must also become a generalist. A more holistic approach will inevitably mean that medical professionals will have to begin to grapple with some very complex social issues. The health professional will have to become a student, gleaning insights from many sources: anthropology, the social sciences and theology.

REFERENCES

Lewis, O (1966) The Culture of Poverty in Lewis, O *La Vida* Random House, New York
McKnight, J (1989) Why Servantshood is Bad *The Other Side* vol 25 no 1, pp38–40
University of the Philippines (1987) Based on a survey of urban poor women, conducted by the University of the Philippines Population Institute

14

Action and Research in Urban Health Development – Progress and Prospects

Marcel Tanner and Trudy Harpham

Urban growth and urbanization will continue in the Third World over the next decades. The complex interactions between political, social and economic factors will strengthen rather than decrease this trend and consequently lead to an even higher degree of segregation in most cities. Thus, the social and economic differentials will be substantial and will be drastically reflected in intra-urban differentials of morbidity and mortality. Working on urban health development, do we have to accept such a bleak outlook and restrict ourselves to reduce some suffering by applying biomedical tools, drugs or vaccines, or intervention packages? There is an alternative urban future which Hardoy et al (1990) describe: 'where government policies become rooted in making best use of local skills, knowledge, culture and resources. This requires that governments turn to the capacities of the people who are already the most active city builders – individual citizens and the community organizations they form'. The attempts to strengthen urban health development processes as outlined in this book match this statement at both the level of implementation and research.

The crucial role of communities emerges at all levels and within each effort of internal or external support of urban health development. Neither the analysis of the determinants of urban health status, nor the consideration of the health care delivery and health promotion system, nor the case studies indicate that a major impact on the health of urban populations and their quality of life can be realized by technical solutions and standardized intervention packages. While the usefulness of biomedical tools is not questioned, the experience summarized in this book not only emphasizes that strategies in public health, environmental sanitation, education and infrastructure support need to be carefully tailored to local conditions, but – more importantly – indicate the importance of considering the demands and felt needs of the different population strata involved. This leads to important implications for urban health research and for the implementation of urban health programmes.

Research should no longer only describe health status, health behaviour and measure health impact, but aim at the measurement and the analysis of risk groups, risk behaviours and risk sites within urban populations which will specifically reveal intra-urban differentials and provide a sound basis for priority setting and planning. On the quantitative side one would like to see a move from the disease/condition based to risk based DALYs (Murray et al 1994) that also incorporate people's perception and ranking of the severity of the conditions. Substantial innovative approaches and numerous studies in different areas are required to pursue this important avenue in public health research. This concept entails as a prerequisite that research approaches move towards systems approaches, ie community based action research processes. Qualitative and quantitative data collection methods coming from the biomedical and social sciences will have to be applied. The static hypothesis is replaced by a dynamic one and the ultimate aim of the research process is change. The scientist still applies empirical principles, but based on quasi-experimental approaches. Given these conditions of research, the researcher always moves on the continuum between operational plausibility and scientific probability, ie needs to take a position as to what extent the decision following any analysis should be based on a probability or a plausibility statement. Once this choice is made together with implementers in the health sector, research can be more effectively translated into public health action.

Studies on determinants of the quality of health care and, consequently, of the health seeking behaviour of an urban population, represent a priority area of research that is again closely linked to direct application. The perceived quality of care by users and non-users of any level and type of service compared to the technical quality of care will help us to understand the complex user-provider patterns in different urban settings and will lead to rational coverage plans for urban health services. The lack of a specific chapter on health seeking behaviour and the scarce data on it in all the chapters and case studies underline the need for further research in this area which would be an ideal topic for community based action research as emphasized above.

The process of priority setting is another important area where there is a substantial research need. Although several methods have been proposed and are discussed in the chapters of Tanner and Harpham, and Seager, there is a need to comparatively evaluate the different approaches with regard to feasibility and efficiency during routine application, ie within the regular planning process within municipalities or urban districts or regions. A careful analysis of costs, the possibilities of financing and of resource allocation within the urban sector must complement research on priority setting. In addition, it represents an important area for research and evaluation. The discussion and the operational framework provided in the chapter by Thomas and McPake for health and environmental services will hopefully stimulate relevant research and guide the evaluation of urban health development programmes.

Turning to urban health development programmes, they will also have to establish methods and procedures to monitor people's perceptions and demand patterns in terms of both health service delivery and health promotion activities. As outlined in several chapters and revealed in the research needs, we face an important lack of the application of methods and procedures to 'listen to communities' (Salmen 1987, Vlassoff 1992) and therefore often plan activities without considering fully the community components. This demands a critical review of the different levels of implementation arrangements of urban health development initiatives:

• the type of project/programme;
• the level of integration within existing structures; and
• the collaboration and partnerships established which require particular attention.

The past experience in urban health initiatives is primarily based on **projects**, ie comparatively short term arrangements (≤ five years) that are linked with existing structures, but not often truly integrated. The project based approach is often used among bilateral and multilateral donors as well as NGOs during initial stages and much emphasis is put on reaching objectives, testing and validating approaches, without aiming specifically at sustainability. Longer term involvement and commitments in the range between five to ten years that aim at launching and maintaining health development processes require a **programme based** approach. A programme is seen in this context as an integrated component within the health plan of a municipality or an urban district or region. The programme is implemented within the existing structures (governmental, NGO, private) by the available staff, but often reinforced by short term or even a few long term experts. Any external support represents assistance to an existing structure.

The discussion of the possibilities and degree of integration of an urban health programme or component into existing structures should be guided by an analysis of decision making within the municipality and its health department or sector. The level of decentralization and, thus, the levels where responsibility and authority are assigned, will indicate how a programme can be implemented and sustained. These elements have been well described in the chapter by Lorenz and Garner. It is evident that a decentralized management of the health system based on the health district concept is feasible and preferable in urban settings, as it allows health plans to be tailored to the needs of particular areas within a large city. In addition, the planners and decision makers are closer to their communities which again would allow them to take into account more effectively the populations' perceptions and expectations. This, in turn, is a basis for the democratization of the public services as promoted in the chapter by Lorenz and Garner.

The type and nature of the network of internal and external partnerships are closely related to the level of integration. As clearly demonstrated in the case studies, NGOs play a key role at the interface between communities and the municipal governments. NGOs not only assure the communication, the expression of demand to local and national decision makers, but they also are in an excellent position to identify existing initiatives at the community level. Having picked them up, they can also act as a catalyst to assist these initiatives to succeed or to assure the dissemination of the experience and its application elsewhere.

The case studies illustrating the development of drug stores and a simple insurance scheme for the slum populations in Manila are relevant examples in this context (see Boxes 13.1 and 13.2 in the chapter by Duncan and Auer). The schemes initially developed in one slum area of Manila were adopted nationally.

So far we have mainly referred to international NGOs. However, in order to render NGOs even more effective and more integrated, one would like to see that local and national NGOs are strengthened. It is well understood that such national NGOs can, even should, be assisted by international NGOs and other agencies. Impressive steps in this direction have been summarized in a recent book on funding and supporting community initiatives with regard to housing and living conditions (Arossi et al 1994). The approaches illustrated, discussed and proposed in this book are of great relevance for ongoing and future urban health development programmes.

International bilateral and multilateral donors will continue to play an important role in supporting priority action and research in the urban sector, particularly with regard to urban health. The relevant chapters summarizing the experience from bodies such as the World Bank, WHO, UNICEF, USAID and GTZ show remarkably convergent trends. Most of the agencies started with smaller, well defined, but weakly integrated projects and moved towards the programme based approach emphasizing interdisciplinary action. In addition, most emphasize the role of NGOs and actively collaborate with them in their programmes. Moreover, all the agencies point to the need to reach an optimal balance between the public and private sector with regard to the provision and the financing of health care and health promotion services. The evaluation of the first five to ten years of experience of their urban health and development programmes will soon be due and we see this moment as an important milestone to review policies, concepts and strategies that have guided these institutions together with their partners in the South. A careful analysis of this experience will be crucial to maintain awareness of urban issues and to secure some of the funds required to realize the new urban future (Hardoy et al 1990).

We believe that all the chapters have clearly emphasized that 'deprofessionalization of the health services is the single most important step in raising health standards in the Third World' (Djukanovic and Mach 1975). This not only leads to the conclusion that urban health problems are too large, and the underlying determinants are too complex, for them to be managed by ministries of health alone, but strongly emphasizes the intersectoral, collaborative arrangements that need to be established within a city and between the different groups of interested parties that provide internal and external assistance. Clearly, the problems that we face in urban health development are of a multidisciplinary nature; however, they can only be tackled through an interdisciplinary approach as we aim at transdisciplinary solutions ie solutuions in which the separation and respective contributions of the single disciplines are not visible or relevant due to the fact that emphasis is placed on solving problems within the 'transdiscipline' of urban development. It is this concept that the present book also aimed at promoting, in order to face the challenge that 'urbanization...will become one of the most critical development issues in the years ahead' (Chalker in Harris 1992) and to contribute to the new urban future.

REFERENCES

Arossi, S Bombarolo, F Hardoy, J Mitlin, D Coscio, L Satterthwaite, D (1994) *Funding Community Initiatives* Earthscan, London

Djukanovic, V and Mach, E (1975) Alternative Approaches to Meeting Basic Health Needs in Developing Countries in: *Health by the People* Newell, K (ed) World Health Organization, Geneva

Hardoy, J Cairncross, S Satterthwaite, D (1990) *The Poor Die Young: Housing and Health in Third World Cities* Earthscan, London

Harris, N (1992) *Cities in the 1990s: The Challenge for Developing Countries* UCL Press, London

Murray, C Lopez, A Jamison, D (1994) The Global Burden of Disease in 1990: Summary Results, Sensitivity Analysis and Future Directions *Bulletin of the World Health Organization* 72, pp495–509

Salmen, L (1987) *Listen to the People: Participant-Observer Evaluation of Development Projects* Oxford University Press, Oxford

Vlassoff, C (1992) Listening to People: Improving Disease Control using Social Science Approaches *Trans Royal Society of Tropical Medicine and Hygiene* 86 pp465–466

Index